Student Nurse Assignments

By

Cordelia Maison

Version 1.0
Published 10th July 2014

Disclaimer and Terms of Use Agreement

The author of this book has used her best efforts in preparing this book. The author makes no representation or warranties with respect to the accuracy or completeness of the contents of this book. The information contained in this book is strictly for educational purposes. The author shall in no event be held liable to any party for any direct, indirect, punitive, special, incidental or other consequential damages arising directly or indirectly from any use of this material which is provided without warranty.

About the author

I'm a forty something year old mother of 6 children. My rather colourful life began in the sixties in Hertfordshire, born into a working class family of mixed heritage. My grandmother on my father's side was Russian, my grandfather Greek; on my mother's side were a mix of British and Irish heritage.

My parents separated when I was only a few years old. The ripple effects from the dissolution of the stereotype perfect family were huge leading down paths many will never experience, that said the lessons and experiences encountered are what make me who I am today. The net result was that I left school having just turned sixteen with only two GCE's and two CSE's to my name. I was always of the belief that I was not college material and so resigned myself to a working life in a factory environment following in my mother's footsteps. After only a year I came to realise that I was living a life that society expected from people with backgrounds like mine, my mind on the other hand was opposing this stereotype. Subsequent years have seen me progress through college and university while bringing up my six children.
In my early forties my mother passed away after a gruelling illness which took a heavy toll on my

family. Evaluating my life I realised change was the only way I could feel I wasn't just letting years slip by needlessly. That's when I came up with the most bizarre idea of how to change my life. I needed to step out of my comfort zone to feel alive. As a child growing up I remember being asked by different people "what do you want to be when you grow up?" There never seemed to be much choice, teacher, fireman, nurse.... the one thing I knew was that I never wanted to be nurse. In my young mind nurses were on par with waitresses and for reasons I did not understand at the time I saw nurses, waitresses etc as little more than servants unappreciated, overworked, unhappy and unrewarded. Reflecting back I feel my negative outlook on certain professions was based on my observations seeing my mother, grandmother, aunts and self constantly subjected to degradation, particularly by males, but also my role models such as my early year teachers and general society. So, to step out of my comfort zone, to challenge myself, my beliefs, my life, in the midst's of grief I enrolled on a nursing course.

Today I have several years of nursing practice behind me and needless to say I now view nurses, waitresses etc. with a different eye.

Contents

Chapter 1

What is a case study? 11

Chapter 2

What is Patient centred care? 23

Chapter 3

What is a Learning Contract? 35

Chapter 4

What is Communication?.................................46

Chapter 5

What is a Care Study?.....................................57

Chapter 6

What is Group Working? 72

Chapter 7

What is a Learning Contract? 80

Chapter 8

What is a Care Study?.....................................93

Chapter 9

What is Group Working? 109

Chapter 10

What is a reflective essay?..............................120

Chapter 11

What is a narrative essay? 135

Introduction

After graduating from university I began working as a qualified adult nurse in the UK. I was fortunate that I found work instantly and my nursing knowledge has gone from strength to strength since. My journey here was hard as I had missed a portion of compulsory UK schooling while living in the USA and generally being a bad student preferring to skip lessons, as this was much easier than having to deal with people. In my adult life against all the odds I have managed to successfully complete a nursing course and now practice professionally as a qualified adult nurse.

This book is a compilation of some nursing assignments I wrote. I wanted to share my work as evidence that with determination, even lacking formal qualifications anyone can achieve their goals. The assignments contained within this book are registered on a plagiarism database through the university that I studied with. The contents of this book are not endorsed by any professional body and serve only as an example based on my own experience and knowledge. Any official guidance/instruction should be followed and this book used only for background information.

By reading this book I hope it may inspire someone to keep trying. Grades obtained are not included as these assignments serve only to demonstrate writing style and types of assignments today's nursing students can expect.

I would like to thank my family for their support during my studies, without whom I would not be where I am today.

How to use this book

Each chapter of this book represents an assignment. The assignments are published in their original form as submitted to the university. A prologue has been provided at the start of each chapter to explain what the assignment is based on and its relation to healthcare.

Chapter 1

What is a Case Study?

A process or record of research into the development of a particular person, group, or situation over a period of time (Google, 2014). Case studies enable the student to become actively involved in the learning process (Bonwell and Eison, 1991, Sivan et al, 2000). A case study is a student centred activity that enables the student to demonstrate knowledge based theory drawing on experience gained while in a placement setting. According to Fry et al (1999) case studies are complex examples which give an insight into the context of a problem as well as illustrating the main point.

Professional Practice in Nursing
Case Study

My case study is centred on a male patient (patient X) post stroke presenting with dementia. The purpose of this study is to look at an aspect of care delivery and how it was managed. I will be focusing on feeding. The areas I will be looking at are the importance of nutritional status, dietary care plan and method of delivery and management. In order to understand the delivery and management of this issue I will be looking at some aspects of the Mental Capacity Act 2005 and the Nursing and Midwifery Council (NMC) code of standards and the National Institute for Clinical Excellence (NICE) guidelines. A brief profile of patient X is contained within appendix A.

Patient X was admitted onto a mental assessment ward as his behaviour had deteriorated to a point that was not maintainable at home. Observation of patient X revealed a quiet man who would become agitated and aggressive when personal car was offered. When help with personal hygiene or food was presented to patient X he would simply refuse by becoming physically and audibly aggressive. Patient X's wife was unhappy with the condition of her husband and insisted that staff wash, shave and feed him; Mrs X initially refused to believe that her husband was uncooperative and felt that his deteriorating hygiene and continued weight loss was due to staff neglect. A multi disciplinary team (MDT) meeting was held with Mr and Mrs X present and a care plan agreed. Mr X although present was unable to participate in the meeting as the dementia meant he no longer spoke, although he would smile when his wife was present and generally be more cooperative when she was there.

One of the major concerns for Mr X was his 20% weight loss over the last few months. A dietician was consulted to review Mr X and several food and fluid supplements were added to Mr X's drug chart to be given at every meal time. The problem now was not what care was needed, but how was it going to be delivered as Mr X frequently refused to eat or drink anything? Through trial and error staff found that Mr X would eat and drink of his own free will once he had tasted that initial food or drink in his mouth. Getting that initial spoonful of food or sip of fluid into Mr X's mouth was the hard part, as he would start kicking, punch, scream and refuse to open his mouth. It was not unusual for it to take several hours to try and persuade Mr X to eat.

As Mr X was mentally incapacitated his consent to being feed was not obtainable. Three members of staff would assist Mr X to be fed. Two members of this three man team would each hold one of Mr X's arms and or legs while the other one would explain to Mr X that they are going to feed him. The purpose of restraining Mr X was firstly to enable Mr X to be fed and secondly to protect the feeder from being hit by Mr X. Once that first spoon of food was sensed by Mr X on his lips he would open his mouth and then the two supporting members of staff were able to let go of Mr X's arms and or legs and he would then either feed himself or allow the other member of staff to feed him with no further resistance. This was seen as acting in the patients' best interest.

Consent was not obtained from Mr X due to mental incapacity. The Mental Capacity Act 2005 (MCA) states that anyone acting on behalf of an incapacitated person must do so according to the prior wishes of the incapacitated person, or if these are not known then you must act in the best interest of the incapacitated person in the least intrusive way (Great Britain, The Mental Capacity Act 2005). Although Mr X was unable to give initial consent to being fed his cooperation to eat once he had tasted the first spoon of food implied consent, and therefore his wife and the healthcare officials were acting in his best interest when using the restraint.

How necessary was it to feed Mr X and in this way? It has been known for a long time that nutrition is an important factor in maintaining a healthy body that leads to better healthcare outcomes (Coxal, 2008). Age Concern, in their campaign "Hungry to be Heard 2008", state that malnourished elderly people are more prone to mental impairment which can lead to longer hospital stays and increased mortality. Nutrition is recognised as an important part of health by the National Institute for Clinical Excellence (NICE) who have said that every patient on their first hospital visit inpatient or outpatient should have a nutritional status evaluation carried out (NICE, 2006). The Department of Health have their own campaign called "Essence of Care 2001" – which provides support measures to raise quality for patients that includes nutritional status. Although Mr X's clinical diagnoses is not curable it is possible to improve his quality of life by improving his nutritional status, this is acting in Mr X's best interest. Failing to feed Mr X would be an act of omission on the part of the professional care giver as he is unable to perform the act of eating without prompt due to mental incapacity.

The delivery of care afforded to Mr X could be seen to be abuse as the restraining techniques would amount to assault if used on a capacitated individual in the same way. To protect both Mr X and the healthcare professionals involved in his care it is paramount that the care plan is included in Mr X's medical notes together with a journal of daily care given to Mr X, including how the care was delivered, what the outcome of the care was and how Mr X responded to the care. Keeping clear and accurate nursing records is part of the Royal College of Nursing code of practice (RCN, 2008).

It could easily become routine to restrain Mr X to start feeding him without first asking him if he is hungry, or if he would like to feed himself, or would he like some help, giving him the choice. Although it had been agreed that Mr X could be restrained it was only acceptable to use the restraint if Mr X was not eating enough to sustain a healthy diet and only if he became physically aggressive when the health care providers were trying to assist with feeding him. The use of restraint as routine procedure would be abuse and not acting in Mr X's best interest. Regular MDT meetings with Mr X's wife were held to review the care being delivered, this helped to make sure that the care being provided was relevant to Mr X based on how he is and not on how he was. By holding regular MDT meetings staff were acting as a team making sure that Mr X was being treated individually and that he was their first priority which is part of the remit of the RCN (RCN, 2008).

This case study highlighted to me some very important issues. The importance of putting the patient first, how to address issues of consent while acting in the patient best interest, and how legislation enables healthcare professionals to treat patients in a legally safe way, protecting patient best interest and professional liability, provided of course, that the legislation and professional codes have been followed. It is important to be aware of the professional code of conduct for nurses and midwifes as it acts as a safe guard for both the patient and the nurse practitioner through maintaining standards by following codes of practice. Following the legislation, professional codes of standards, acting in best interest of patients and being aware of relevant issues and campaigns means that the professional healthcare providers, in this case the nurse practitioners are acting in accordance with their profession as a professional.

Appendix
Patient Profile

Male
76 Years Old
Dementia
Incontinent urine/faeces

HISTORY

Sep 2005	Fall
2005	Pneumothorax
22 Sep 2005	Pulmonary Embolus
26 Sep 2005	Pulmonary Embolus
Dec 2005	Stroke
Dec 2005	Headaches worsening
Jan 2006	Intracerebral haemorrhage
6 Feb 2006	MRI – still bleeding
10 Feb 2006	Intracerebal haemorrhage
31 Feb 2006	x-ray haematoma left temporal – old infarct
Feb 2006	MRSA
2006	Collapsed lung
2006	Pulmonary embolism
29 Jun 2008	MRSA positive groin, wound left elbow, nose

This admission

Aggressive, agitated, screaming, wandering, underweight, poor eater, 20% weight loss

Drugs

Name	To Treat	Comment
Haloperidol	Aggression	No effect
Promazine	Aggression	No effect
Quefiapine		25mg x2 daily (No effect)
Carbamazedine	Mood stabiliser	100mgs daily
Diazepam	Anxiety	As required
Risperodone		(not depressed)
Calogen	Food supplement	3x daily
Ensure	Food supplement	3x daily
Fybogel	Constipation	As required

Reference

Age Concern (2006), Hungry to be Heard. Available at: http://www.ageconcern.org.uk/AgeConcern/ Documents/Hungry_to_be_Heard_ August 2006.pdf, (Accessed 28th August 2008)

Bonwell C C and Eison J A (1991) Active Learning: Creating Excitement in the Classroom, ASHE-ERIC Higher Education Report No. 1. The George Washington University, School of Education and Human Development, Washington, DC.

Coxal (2008), Applying the key principles of nutrition to nursing practice, Nursing Standard Vol 22(36) pp 44-48, EBSCO host research database – Academic Search Elite [Online], Available at http://0-web.ebscohost.com.brum.beds.ac.uk/ehost/pdf ?vid=4andhid=115andsid=29e27cc1-712d-4713-96d6-fd739c89f419%40sessionmgr108 (Accessed: 28th August 2008)

Department of Health (2001), Essence of Care, Available at: http://www.dh.gov.uk/en/publicationsand statistics/publications/publicationspolicyandgu idance/DH_4005475 (Accessed: 28th August 2008)

Fry H, Ketteridge S and Marshall S (1999) A Handbook for Teaching and Learning in Higher Education, Kogan Page, Glasgow, pp408

Google (2014) Available at: https://www.google.co.uk/?gws_rd=ssl#q=what+is+a+case+study

Great Britain Mental Capacity Act 2005: Elizabeth II Chapter 9. (2005) London: The Stationery Office

National Institute for Health and Clinical Excellence (2006), Nutrition support in adults: Clinical Guideline 32. Available at: http://www.nice.org.uk/nicemedia/pdf/cg032 fullguidelineappendices.pdf, (Accessed: 28th August 2008)

Nursing and Midwifery Council (2008), The Code: Standards of Conduct, Performance and Ethics for Nurses and Midwives, NMC, London

Sivan A, Wong Leung R, Woon C and Kember D (2000) An Implementation of Active Learning and its Effect on the Quality of Student Learning

Innovations in Education and Training
International. Vol. 37 No 4 pp381-389

Chapter 2

What is Patient centred care?

Patient centred care supports active involvement of patients and their families in the design of new care models and in decision-making about individual options for treatment. Putting the patient foremost through communication, discussion of treatment options, potential outcomes and psychological effects allows and empowers the patient to make choices about their healthcare. (Nursing Standard, 2014)

Patient Centred Care
Study

This study aims to identify the care needs of a patient. My remit is to look at the care given to this individual and how the care was delivered according to the patients' needs reflecting the patient's personality while maintaining the patient's best interest. The aspect of care that I am going to look at is personal care, washing and dressing. For the purpose of this study I will not be going into how consent was gained or what medication my patient was on.

The patient I have chosen for this study is an elderly man in his seventies with a history of strokes leading to vascular dementia. Before having a stroke this gentleman was an active man keen on gardening who kept an allotment and walked his dogs every day. My chosen patient has been married for forty plus years and smoked all of his adult life.

Over the last three years this gentleman's (Mr X) health had been failing after a fall in a hospital car park while visiting an elderly relative. The fall resulted in injury to Mr X's ribs, probably the cause of his pneumothorax (collapsed lung), later in the same month Mr X had two separate incidents of pulmonary embolus (blood clot in the lung) and then within three months suffered a stroke. Over the course of the next two months Mr X had a further intracerebal haemorrhage which bleed for a number of weeks, a further pneumothorax and pulmonary embolism. During this period of hospital visits Mr X also contracted MRSA.

The net result of all of these health problems was that Mr X's personality and behaviour began to change. Within three years Mr X had lost almost half of his original body weight. The strokes caused Mr X to develop vascular dementia, the cause of his behavioural changes. Mrs X found it difficult to cope with her husband's agitated and aggressive state, he would scream uncontrollably for no apparent reason and often wander off with no idea of where he was or why he had gone. Mr X was admitted onto an assessment ward so that health professionals could work out what his medical and social needs were, and how these could be facilitated.

Mr X is a frail elderly man who was resistive to being washed or dressed. The health care professionals were faced with washing and dressing a man who did not want to be touched or moved and would not communicate verbally with anyone. Once washed and dressed Mr X would appear more content muttering and even smiling at people he came into contact with. It was decided that daily washing and dressing was in Mr X's best interest to avoid further health problems and to help maintain his pre illness routine.

Every morning myself and a HCA would go into Mr X's room to wash and dress him ready for breakfast. Even though Mr X did not speak we would say good morning to him using his first name and explain why we were there and ask if it was OK to help him to get washed and dressed. Sometimes Mr X would be fast asleep so we would say audibly that we will let him sleep a little longer and be back in a bit. If Mr X was awake we would continue with assisting Mr X to wash and dress. Mr X was incontinent of urine and faeces and wasn't catheterised. Filing to wash Mr X would not be in his best interest as lying in his own urine and faeces could cause Mr X further health problems such as skin break down, at best not washing would/could cause Mr X to be uncomfortable and cold. Mr X would often become aggressive when staff were attending to his incontinence, while this part of his personal care was taking place he would scream, hit and kick, it was often necessary for another HCA to be called in to help by holding his arms and or legs while he was cleaned up. Generally after this part of the care was given Mr X would become more cooperative. Even though morning care was delivered every day, every day the care givers would say who they were and what they were there to do.

It was my experience when assisting Mr X that he would re-act differently depending upon how the care was delivered. Difference in how care is administered and its effectiveness has been recognised by the Department of Health who acknowledge dementia as one of the most major diseases set to continue to rise over the next 20 plus years, so have published a plan to improve care (Department of Health, 2008). All the care givers provided Mr X with good care as far as making sure he was clean, dry and comfortable but the real difference came with those care givers who personalised the care. For instance, Mr X's bedroom window opened out onto a rarely used footpath, there was no real need to close the curtains as the likely hood of someone seeing in were very remote. I noted that when care givers acknowledged the open curtain and so closed it before continuing care, Mr X would still be resistive to the care, but, when the care giver closed the curtain and told Mr X that they were closing the curtain so that they could give him a wash he would become less resistive to the care. "Well intentioned care needs knowledge" (Nazarko, 2008) the former example illustrates how a different approach to care can lead to a more positive outcome, this particular care giver had researched dementia so had a better understanding as to why dementia patients behave in certain ways, this knowledge meant she was able to adapt her care in order to achieve the best possible outcome for Mr X, which in this instance was to maintain his hygiene with his cooperation.

Dressing Mr X was routine, he only had a small selection of clothes in his wardrobe it was easier to put jogging bottoms and sweatshirt on Mr X than to put on shirt and formal trousers. Dressing Mr X was always a battle but an accepted one whereby Mr X would resist and the care givers would compensate. Distraction seemed to work best with one person delegated the task of putting the item on, eg put the jogging bottoms on while the other care giver brushed his teeth or his hair. I thought this was clever until I witnessed a care giver with a different approach. Allowing Mr X to brush his own teeth gained a lot more cooperation from him, the care giver would acknowledge Mr X's effort and praise it and if necessary offer help to do the bits he was having difficulty with, such as getting a cup of water so that he could rinse his mouth out. When it came to dressing I found that when Mr X was given the choice of deciding what to wear, he became more manageable by being less resistive to the care being administered. Mr X could not speak but his resistance to having a sweatshirt put on, compared to his cooperation in having a shirt put on was his way of communicating his preference of attire. According to Hobson (2008), people with dementia use body language, in particular agitation, restlessness or aggression as a means of communication.

After reading Mr X's hospital notes and speaking to his wife I found out that Mr X used to be a keen gardener and kept an allotment. The next time that I was delegated as Mr X's named carer for the day I spoke about gardening and the rewards of growing your own vegetables, Mr X was not able to contribute to the conversation but there was a notable difference in how Mr X responded to care, he still resisted but not with the same amount of aggression I had come to expect.

There has been a study done that looked at the difference between behaviours of people with dementia during the period when morning care was administered. One group of elderly people with dementia were given their normal morning care and the other group of people were given their morning care, but with instruction of personalising the care by using the patients' name, acknowledging their emotions, responding to their actions or behaviours, being patient and respectful. It was found that the group of people who had their care personalised exhibited less agitation and aggressive behaviour than the group receiving their normal morning care. (Weert et al 2006)

Mr X has been married for forty plus years and always been the provider for his family. Now Mr X is resigned to being cared for by strangers. The morning care is delivered by different people, it could be that someone different is carrying out the personal care every day of the week. Most people would respect the wishes of an able person but for some reason act differently when some ones capacity to communicate diminishes. Mr X is still a proud man with feelings and some understanding. Although it may be difficult to understand what Mr X is trying to communicate it became obvious that when Mr X's dignity and honour where respected by including and enabling him to contribute to his own care he became more cooperative. The act of acknowledgement as when telling Mr X that you had closed the curtains thus maintaining his dignity led to a more positive response. Once Mr X's behaviours were understood it became much easier to administer his care. Client centred approaches to care enable individualised measures of function to take place which basically means that what works for one patient is individualised to them in order to achieve, in this case, the best possible quality of life with as much input and or participation from the patient as is possible maximising their potential (Donnelly et al 2004).

My study has looked at the behaviour of Mr X during morning care and compared it depending on the approaches used to carry out the care. The care Mr X received was compared to a study into behaviour versus care of people with dementia. It is very easy to focus on tasks and not people when there is so much to be completed within a time frame, but when care is personalised it has the effect of giving people the feeling of self worth and that sense of identity, our own uniqueness. My study has shown that when identity is striped it can become harder to treat the person. It is unconceivable to treat a disease effectively without knowing the disease how it behaves and interact; equally you cannot treat a person effectively without knowing the person how they behave and interact this is what is known as person centred care (Strokes 2005).

Reference

Department of Health (2008), Transforming the quality of dementia care: consultation on a National Dementia Strategy, Available at: http://www.dh.gov.uken/Consultations/Close dconsultations/DH_085570. (Accessed 14th September 2008)

Donnelly, En, Hall, Alford, Giachino, Norton, Kerr (2004), Client-Centred assessment and identification of meaningful treatment goals for individuals with spinal cord injury, Spinal Cord Vol 42 pp302-307 – ESBSO host research database CINAHL [Online], Available at: http://0-web.ebscohost.com.brum.beds.ac.uk/ehost/pdf?vid=6andhid=5andsid=29d183b0-d1f5-4229-a828-e12a90126747%40sessionmgr2. (Accessed: 17th September 2008)

Weert, Janssen, Dulmen, Spreeuwenberg, Bensing, Ribbe (2006), Nursing assistants' behaviour during morning care: effects of the implementation of snoezelen, integrated in 24-hour dementia care, Journal of advanced nursing Vol 53(6) pp 656-668, EBSCO host research database CINAHL [Online]. Available at: http://0-web.ebscohost.com.brum.beds.ac.uk/ehost/pdf

?vid=6andhid=7andsid=ff91bbb8-3c99-4964-8bfa-abbd049b6172%40SRCSMI. (Accessed: 14th September 2008)

Nazarko (2008), Dressed to impress: dressing in dementia, Nursing and Residential Care Vol 10(8) pp401-403 – EBSCO host research database – CINAHL [Online] Available at: http://0-web.ebscohost.com.brum.beds.ac.uk/ehost/pdf ?vid=3andhid=5andsid=e3ec08c2-d6c4-4b28-8c4e-c1af0cdd8c9b%40sessionmgr2. (Accessed: 14th September 2008)

Hobson (2008), Understanding dementia: developing person-centred communication, British Journal of Healthcare Assistants Vol 2(4) pp 162-164 – ESBSO host research database CINAHL [Online] Available at: http://0-web.ebscohost.com.brum.beds.ac.uk/ehost/pdf ?vid=9andhid=5andsid=29d183b0-d1f5-4229-a828-e12a90126747%40sessionmgr2. (Accessed: 17th September 2008)

Nursing Standard (2014) Promoting Excellence in Nursing Care, Available at: http://rcnpublishing.com/page/ns/students/clinical-placements/patientcentred-care (Accessed 26th June 2014)

Stokes (2005), Enhancing Practice, person centred care for residents with dementia,

Nursing and Residential Care Vol 7(3) pp 109 –
ESBSO host research database CINAHL [Online}
Available at: http://0-
web.ebscohost.com.brum.beds.ac.uk/ehost/pdf
?vid=10andhid=5andsid=29d183b0-d1f5-4229-
a828-e12a90126747%40sessionmgr2. (Accessed:
17th September 2008)

Chapter 3

What is a Learning Contract?

A learning contract is one method of implementing the concepts of self-directed learning. Goals and Objectives: The overall goal of the learning contract is to allow the student to take responsibility for his/her own learning. A learning need is the gap between where you are and where you want to be.

Learning Contract
Explore legal issues in health care

- To become aware of the Mental Health Act 1983 and the Mental Capacity Act 2005
- To understand the purpose of the Acts
- To become aware of the contents of the Acts
- To understand the rights of people lacking mental capacity
- To understand how to determine if someone lacks mental capacity

- To understand my role as a nurse caring for people with limited mental capacity
- To expand my awareness of difference/vulnerability in society
- To empathise with people lacking mental capacity

In order to succeed in achieving my learning need of becoming aware of legal issues within health care, I have had to first narrow down the subject and have chosen to focus on two act "The Mental Health Act 1983" and "The Mental Capacity Act 2005".

My research started with the "Crown" legislation, the Acts themselves and supporting documents that outline the content of these Acts. Medical Journals specialising in mental health, community nursing and ethics have also proved to be an invaluable source of information. The aforementioned sources of information were useful for covering the theory but it was my placement experiences that really cemented the knowledge by applying theory to practice. My placements have included a stroke ward in a NHS hospital setting, a dementia assessment ward with a NHS trust and a working farm for people with learning disabilities. I have also used the internet where I discovered Mind, a charity whose ethos is to try and improve the lives of people affected by mental distress by raising awareness, campaigning and educating the public and government on issues faced by people affected by mental health issues. Together the above sources of information have helped in providing a diverse knowledge base to help achieve my learning need.

The Mental Health Act 1983 (MHA) covers four categories of mental disorders being mental illness, severe mental impairment with aggressive/irresponsible conduct, mental impairment and psychopathic disorders (Mind 2006). The purpose of the Act is to allow for the confinement and treatment in a hospital for people with a mental disorder. The criteria for confinement vary slightly between people with/without involvement in criminal proceedings.

The MHA is split into many sections each section identifies a specific criterion and states the policy to follow in each case. Involuntary confinement usually requires that two doctors confirm the mental disorder and that the confinement is for the protection and safety of the public and person with the mental disorder. The application for section would normally come from a social worker or nearest relative of the person with the mental disorder. Confinement has statutory time limits which can be reviewed/renewed if the health officials or nearest relative feels is necessary. The person with the mental disorder is not powerless and can apply to the Mental Health Review Tribunal (MHRT) for discharge (Mind 2006).

People with a mental disorder involved in criminal proceedings can be sectioned in much the same way as an individual not involved with criminal proceedings. The main difference is that the two qualifying doctors who confirm the mental disorder must agree that treatment will alleviate or prevent further deterioration of the person with the mental disorder. It is also possible to apply for a restriction order/hospital order for those at risk from self harm. Discharge can be sanctioned by the Home Secretary or MHRT (Mind 2006).

Most people in hospital with a mental disorder are voluntary (informal) patients with only 15% of these under section (formal) (Mind 2006). Patients have the right to information on their section, right of appeal, and consent to treatment and correspondence rules. Health authorities have a legal duty to provide care for patients detained after section has expired and not to charge for this care.

The "Mental Capacity Act 2005" (MCA) is based on the Law Commission Report 231 published February 1995 to clarify unclear law. The act replaces part 7 of MHA and all of the "Attorney Act 1985". The MCA covers decisions making for incapacitated people by attorneys, court deputies or procedure when attorney and deputy not put in a place, it is the first time in 47 years that someone also can consent to treatment through a power of attorney or deputy assigned by a court (Crown 2005, Griffith 2006).

There are three parts to the MCA, defining a person who lacks capacity with the help of a checklist and a code of practice, creation of "Court of Protection" and protection of human right (Crown 2005). The MCA introduces a framework to determine capacity that health officials must adhere to (Griffith 2006).

The MCA starts by presuming capacity unless proven otherwise this is key to autonomy, it preserves the "European Convention on Human Rights" (ECHR), has statutory safe guards in place to protect against liability for carers whether it is a doctor, social worker or nurse so long as rules have been followed. The criterion for incapacity is stated and a checklist to best interest which courts are bound by. Control of property, financial affairs and health are covered with safe guards in place eg a bankrupt person would not be allowed to take over the financial affairs of a mentally impaired person. Lasing Power of Attorney (LPA) can be appointed with power to refuse life saving medical treatment if that was the incapacitated persons wish prior to incapacitation. The MCA has to place rules that must be followed by the LPA. Courts can only force treatment on a patient while a dispute is resolved. Decision making must be given to the patient where ever possible and again there are procedures to follow to allow for this. If the incapacity is temporary then where ever possible decisions must be left until capacity returns (Crown 2005, Griffith 2006).

The MCA allows decisions to be made in advance of incapacity providing that at the time of making the decision the person was capable of doing so, however, this must be of a legal nature e.g. euthanasia is not permitted and care is only allowed to be refused or discontinued, stipulating the type of treatment preferred is for health professionals to decide. There are procedures with the MCA that must be followed to allow for the advance decision to be made (Griffith 2006). Advanced decisions allow for the autonomy of an individual to be upheld even after they become mentally incapacitated.

Another key element of the act is that it includes all mentally impaired people those with drink, drug, head injury, delirium and medical conditions such as dementia, stroke and people with learning disabilities (Griffith 2006). The MCA states incapacity as "an impairment of, or disturbance in the functioning of, the mind or brain". (Great Britain, The Mental Capacity Act 2005)

Compulsory treatment can be administered in the community by applying for a Community Treater Order (CTO) which came into effect in July 2007. Community treatment orders are an amendment to the MHA. For a CTO to be sanctioned the patient must have been previously sectioned against consent (Butcher 2007, English 2006).

The purpose of the MHA and the MCA are to protect people with mental impairment and the public from harm by making available treatment for the mental impairment individual while maintaining their autonomy as much as is possible. Working with incapacitated adults in a learning disability environment, on a stroke ward and in a dementia unit demonstrated to me how vulnerable mentally impaired people are. I have witnessed how fatigue and frustration/depression in stroke patients can lead to a patient refusing treatment even though their dream is to make a full recovery. I have witnessed learning disability clients becoming more confident and enjoying their lives with encouragement and support from others giving them more autonomy over their lives. I have also witnessed dementia at its worst with the sufferer convinced that their medication is an attempted of murder by the health professional and that the health care assistant (HCA) is their devoted wife ready to take them home, clearly this later type of individual would be at risk of harming themselves and or the public if someone did not take the decision to confine them for their own safety.

This learning contract has highlighted the need for me to look beyond what my eyes see and question the motives. While working on a dementia ward I was concerned that patients' wishes were not being respected. My naiveties saw a patient who did not want to get up, washed, dressed and have breakfast as a form of bullying by health care officials. By reading about the MCA and MHA alongside journal reports and questioning staff while on placement, I have been able to understand that the firm action of staff regarding the dementia patient were being carried out in the patients' best interest, as the purpose is to maintain skin integrity, prevent depression and keep the patient nourished etc. I have learnt that your eyes are only one source of evidence and that it is vital to observe, analysing by looking at the situation from both a patient and health professional perspective. Questioning reason for action can address immediate concerns and is in the best interest of both myself and the patient, e.g. if my patient was being bullied then I would have a professional obligation to that patient to report it as stated in the Nursing and Midwifery Council code of professional conduct point 2.5 says "you must report to a relevant person or authority, at the earliest possible time, an conscientious objection that may be relevant to your professional practice. You must continue to provide care to the best of your ability until alternative arrangements are implemented" (NMC 2004). Researching medical conditions, nursing practice and legislation has helped to expand my knowledge and make me more aware of vulnerabilities not always seen. I have been able to identify my need to observe, question and research so that I can improve my own nursing practice without prejudice.

References

Butcher (2007), Controversial Mental Health Bill reaches the finishing line, www.thelancet.com Vol 370 pp 117-118

Crown (2005), Explanatory Notes to Mental Capacity Act 2005 Chapter 9, Available at: http://www.opsi.gov.uk/acts/act2005/en/ukp gaen_20050009_en_1 Accessed 2nd August 2008

English, Hamm, Harrison, Sheather and Sommerville (2006), Ethics briefings, Journal of Medical Ethics Vol 32 pp 619-620

Great Britain, Mental Capacity Act 2005: Elizabeth II Chapter 9, (2005) London: The Stationery Office

Griffith (2006), Making decisions for incapable adults 1: Capacity and the best interest, British Journal of Community Nursing Vol 11(3) pp 119-125

Griffith (2006), Making decisions for incapable adults 2: advanced decisions refusing care, British Journal of Community Nursing Vol 11(4) pp 162-166

Griffith (2006), Making decisions for incapable adults 3: protection, guardians and advocates,

British Journal of Community Nursing Vol 11(5) pp 214-221

Griffith (2006), Making decisions for incapable adults 4: participation in research, British Journal of Community Nursing Vol 11(6) pp 262-265

Mind (2006), The Mental Health Act 1983 an outline guide, available at: http://www.mind.org.uk/NR/rdonlyres/907B B333-FC78-4DD7-98C2-38F2592A41B1/0/MHAoutlineguide2006.pdf Accessed 2nd August 2008

NMC (2004), The NMC code of professional conduct: standards for conduct, performance and ethics, available at http://www.nmc-uk.org/aDisplayDocument.aspx?DocumentID=2 01 Accessed 29th August 2008

Chapter 4

What is Communication?

Communication is the transfer of information between or among people. A basic of good nursing is good communication with patients. Failure to communicate well with a patient right away will destroy the delicate nurse/patient relationship and mean the patient does not trust the nurse. Building relationships is central to nursing work and communication skills can be improved by avoiding jargon and ensuring patients are not labelled.

Communication
Eye Contact

Eye contact is one means of nonverbal communication. This report will look at what eye contact is, what are the beliefs around eye contact, how the beliefs are established, where beliefs originate from, how useful eye contact is in sending and receiving messages and finally to look at eye contact in a healthcare setting. Research used to quantify the report has been gathered using books, journals, the Qur'an and the internet. A reference list is provided at the end of the report. Use of other nonverbal/verbal communication will not be discussed.

Eye contact is something we do every day whether intentionally or not, it is one of many types of nonverbal communication. The difference between feeling embarrassed or rejected can be down to the length of gaze between two people making eye contact. Signalling interest or lack of can be determined by eye contact. Physically as suggested by the two words, eye contact is the meeting of the eyes between two individuals, however, the psychological meaning is not so defined. Eye contact can suggest to the speaker that the audience is interested/disinterested, to the listener honestly/distrust or between the listener/speaker an indication of admiration or hatred. Eye contact signals acknowledgement of presence, involvement and worth (Crawford, 2006) Faulkner 1992). Eye contact works in unison with other verbal/nonverbal factors (Frank 2003), it helps to synchronise conversation.

Western cultures believe lack of eye contact signifies deceit (The Global Deception Research Team 2006, Levin et al 2006) and vice versa good eye contact signifies honesty. Research carried out by (The Global Deception Research Team 2006) set about to study stereotypes about liars to determine if among other criteria eye contact avoidance was typical behaviour of liars.

The study encompassed participant from 75 countries of varying languages. Two groups were established of which one group were given verbal questions and the other group a questionnaire. Culture difference in communication norms suggest that belief stereotypes would vary but interestingly the number one belief across both groups was that eye contact avoidance signalled deceit (The Global Deception Research Team 2006, Levin et al 2006). The Holy Qur'an states

لَخَلْقُ ٱلسَّمَـٰوَٰتِ وَٱلْأَرْضِ أَكْبَرُ مِنْ خَلْقِ ٱلنَّاسِ وَلَـٰكِنَّ أَكْثَرَ ٱلنَّاسِ لَا يَعْلَمُونَ ﴿٥٧﴾

Translated this means "he knoweth the traitor of the eyes, and that which the bosoms hide "(Yusuf 1993). Here we can see that followers of the Qur'an frown upon eye contact between men and women unlike western cultures that interpret eye contact as a social norm with saying like "there's something about his eyes" or "he's making eyes at me". In a study by Park only 10% of participants attributed behaviour as a signal of deceit, 80% of participants discovered deceit over an hour after lie told with 40% of participants discovering the deceit more than seven days later (park 2002). Belief verses actuality is vastly different as shown here.

Knowledge of veracity affects how people see a person's actions (Levin). When it is known that a speaker is lying, eye contact avoidance is sought and confirmed. What is known is that during communication it is natural to look away and make eye contact intermittently. It would be discomforting if a speaker looked at you constantly or the speaker never looked at you. Eye contact/avoidance is a natural part of communication which is independent on message veracity (The Global Deception Research Team 2006).

Gaze times are shown to vary slightly according to the relationship between communicators. Clinician's/layman gaze is less than peer/peer (Turkstra, 2005) in a study of eye contact difference between people with/without traumatic brain injury. One hypothesis for this is that the clinician is able to communicate in a more coherent manner reducing the need for added clues such as pitch, gesture, expression etc. In this group of people some with traumatic brain injury and some without gaze time were similar in both groups and consistent with other studies (Crawford 2006, Turkstra 2005) it is important to note though that the Turkstra study was only to document gaze frequency.

Socially it is deemed that liars should be caught and should feel ashamed about their actions, in this way society vilifies liars. With the aforementioned in mind when an individual appears to withdraw from using eye contact it is conceivable that it can be interpreted as an act of guilt (The Global deception Research Team 2006). If a lie is found out the eye avoidance behaviour is interpreted by the brain as true, unfortunately though it is not fool proof as eye avoidance/contact is also a known natural behaviour in truthful communication (The Global Deception Research Team 2006).

Statistically during verbal communication people look at the face for durations of approximately 3 seconds for about 60% of the time, from this direct contact makes up about 30% of time with durations of approximately one second intervals (Crawford 2006).

The act of looking serves to collect information. Speakers use eye contact as cues e.g. break of eye contact may signal disinterest or termination of conversation (Clark and Krych 2004). If gaze is too long then the listener could interpret this as being spoken at rather than too. In many animals eye contact is perceived as a threat, likewise in human's eye contact of sustained length causes discomfort and feelings of intimidation.

In a health care setting patients are found to disclose more when they feel comfortable and when felt that their problems are of interest (Ann Faulkner 1992). It is known that better communication leads to better health outcomes (McGrath 2007).

The medical interview is a situation whereby it is possible that the patient could feel ignored or that the doctor is disinterested, as part of the interview involves the doctors having to record the interview electronically onto a computer, which by virtue of the task means the doctor, is temporarily disengaged with the patient. A study into the use of the electronic medical record (EMR) during medical interview highlights some positive use of eye contact. Doctors who intermittently turn to use the computer were found to have better eye contact then doctors who spent the entire interview looking/using the computer. The intermittent pauses of computer use allowed time for the patient to ask questions not normally asked about their illness. Health is a private matter whereby a patient may feel uncomfortable disclosing information particularly when eye contact is established. In a practice setting I have noticed that patients tend not to look at you when they feel vulnerable/embarrassed such as when requesting a bed pan or when in some discomfort yet once their needs have been met they are happy to re-establish eye contact. The intermittent EMR use could serve to ease the tension felt by the patient (McGrath 2007).

Good nonverbal communication in a healthcare setting increases patient satisfaction, recall of information doctor has given, better appointment keeping and better compliance to medical instruction. As part of medical training doctors are now offered courses in communication (McGrath 2007).

Emergency health settings place a value on eye contact. A hysterical/distressed person can be calmed by being told to "Look at me". The act of looking helps to restore rationality by forcing the hysterical/distressed individual to re focus (Kidwell 2007).

Eye contact as a standalone means of communication is shown not to be very effective.

Various studies looking at gaze times between people with/without brain injury, about veracity of message and interaction between patient/doctor all show that eye contact/avoidance is consistent. When eye contact is used/interpreted with other forms of communication both verbal/nonverbal it acts to reinforce the message. E.G. a fidgety person showing eye contact could indicate physical discomfort but a fidgety person showing no contact could indicate disinterest in discussion.

I have read about eye contact, behaviour of people with traumatic brain injury against unaffected people, behaviour between peers and between layman/expert, behaviour between liars and truth tellers and between people of different cultures/languages/geographical locations. During university lectures I have been analysing my own eye contact behaviour and have compared it with eye contact between myself and my children when I know they are lying and when they are not and found that my and my children's eye contact behaviour correlate with what I have read. This study has made me rethink my beliefs regarding eye contact and question why people associated eye contact/avoidance as an unspoken message.

References

Yusuf (editor), The Holy Qur'an. 1st edition, place of publication not stated, Wipe International

Clark, Krych (2004) Speaking while monitoring addresses for understanding, Journal of Memory and Language Vol 50(1) pp 62-81

Crawford, Brown and Bohnam (2006), Lynne Wigens (editor) Communication in Clinical Settings 1st edition, Cheltenham UK, Nelson Thornes, Basic interpersonal verbal and non-verbal skills pp 44-45

Faulkner (19992), Effective Interaction with Patient 1st edition, Edinburgh UK, Churchill Livingstone, Non-Verbal Interaction pp 46-47

Feeley, Thomas (2003), To Catch a Liar: Challenges for Research in Lie Detection Training, Journal of Applied Communication Research Vol 31(1) Feb 2003 pp 58-75, EBSCO host research database – Communication and Mass Media

Levin, Asada and Hee (2006). The lying chicken and the gaze avoidant egg: Eye contact deception, and causal order, Southern

Communication Journal, Vol 71(4), Dec 2006, pp
401-411, EBSCO host research database –
PsycINFO

MacMillan (2007), Calm with Eye Contact,
Prevention Magazine Vol 59(9) Sep 2007 pp 152
EBSCO host research database – Academic
search Elite

McCrath, Arar and Pugh (2007). The influence of
electronic medical record usage on nonverbal
communication in the medical interview.
Journal Health Informatics Vol 13(2) Jun 2007 pp
105-118 EBSCO host research database
CASPUR/EJS

Park, Levine, McCornack, Morrison and Ferrara
(2002) pp 144-157, EBSCO host research
database, Communication and Mass Media

The Global Deception Research Team (2006), A
World of Lies, Journal of Cross-Cultural
Psychology Vol 37(1) Jun 2006 pp 60-74, EBSCO
host research database – CASPUR/EJS

Turkstra, University of Wisconsin-Madison
(2005), Looking While Listening and Speaking:
Eye-To-Eye Gaze in Adolescents With and
Without Traumatic Brain Injury, Journal of
Speech, Language and Hearing Research, Vol

48(6), Dec 2005, pp 1429-1441, EBSCO host
research database – PsycINFO

Chapter 5

What is a Care Study?

For this the student is required to identify a nursing problem for the study, formulate a nursing diagnosis and plan of care using research and reflection on the patient perspective.

Care Study
Patient centred care in Acute Care: Incontinence

In this care study I will be looking at an aspect of care given to a patient as part of their care plan. First I will introduce my chose patient and give a brief description containing a little about their background and then reason for admission onto an acute ward. Secondly I shall look briefly at some of the major aspects of care in my patient's care plan and then take one of those aspects and explore the issue further discussing what the problem is, causes and effects of the problem, ways of coping, treatments available and how the care is delivered.

My chosen patient for this care study is a lady who I shall refer to as Freda in her early fifty's. Freda lives with her husband of thirty five years and they have two grown up daughters who live nearby. Freda came into hospital with severe back pain and reduced mobility. On admission Freda was noted to be taking care of her own personal hygiene needs but this was becoming increasingly difficult for her due to the pain she was experiencing in her back. Other exacerbating factors effecting Freda's health were her weight, she has a body mass index greater than thirty, suffers with angina and has a vaginal prolapsed. Prior to admission Freda worked in a charity shop and was a dutiful wife who took pride in taking care of her home and husband.

On admission Freda's care plan highlighted several areas of care that needed to be addressed. The first priority for the health care team was to control Freda's pain with analgesics and to refer Freda to a specialist so that the pain can be investigated. A referral was also sent to the dietician to address Freda's obesity and to the physiotherapist and occupational therapist to address Freda's reduced mobility. Individually each member of the multidisciplinary team introduced themselves to

Freda, explained their role and proposed method of treatment and why this was being offered in opposed to other forms of treatment/therapy available. Freda's agreement to the treatment/therapy was sought and she was given the opportunity to raise any concerns or ask any question she had. As time went on the care plan was revised. Freda became depressed due to the pain and its effect on her diminishing mobility and was now incontinent of urine. I will be discussing urinary incontinence.

The urinary system is controlled mostly by our unconscious nervous system, that is to say it is involuntary. Changes in pressure in the bladder are detected by receptors in the bladder wall receptors in the abdominal muscles detect the stretch of the bladder filling and then relax the sphincter and contract abdominal muscles initiating voiding. As we get older we are able to train our bladders to release voluntarily. Cognitively we reinforce our behaviour in a feedback loop; the voluntary relief of pressure from our bladder is more comfortable than wet legs on an involuntary relief of pressure (Turner et al 1999). Freda is now experiencing the negative feedback of incontinence.

Voiding less than eight times a day and less than two times at night is considered normal (Geriatric Medicine, 2009). Incontinence is when there is an involuntary leakage of urine. Urinary incontinence is sub divided into three main categories, stress, urge and mix. Stress incontinence is when there is leakage on effort for example sneezing (Abrams, 2002). Urge incontinence is when you feel you need to release the urine but there is no or little time between sensing the urge and leakage occurring maybe caused by reduced mobility. Mix incontinence is as the name suggests. There are other causes of urinary incontinence but these can be attributed to either stress or urge, for example an overactive bladder is considered as being urge incontinent (Geriatric Medicine, 2009). There are also medical reasons for being incontinent such as having an urogenital fistulae which is when there is an opening between the bladder and vagina or a vaginal prolapse. Freda is experiencing urge incontinence due to reduced mobility caused by back pain, exacerbated by her medication for her angina and high fluid intake.

There are many causes of incontinence. In the elderly there is evidence to show that there is a higher fall rate which can lead to fractures and even death linked with incontinence (Geriatric

Medicine, 2009).   Thirty percent of falls are thought to be due to or connected with toileting (Thompson, 2007).   Women who have had multiple pregnancies and obese people often go on to experience stress incontinence later in their lives, this is thought to be due to the extra pressure put on the bladder which can cause detrusor muscle damage/weakening (Chiarelli, 1999).   Reduced mobility is another cause of incontinence.   Toileting is something healthy people take for granted, but, when faced with immobility it is easy to see how much strength and flexibility is needed for independent toileting (Earthy, w009).   Dietary intake effects mobility either by volume of fluid intake, alcohol consumption or what we eat.   Incontinence can also be due to an inability to cope with the environment such as difficulty in dressing or toilet being in a very inaccessible place. Incontinence can be aggravated by factors such as cold weather.   Certain drugs can also have effects on incontinence, ACE inhibitors, antipsychotic, benzodiazepines, calcium channel antagonists, diuretics, antimuscarinic drugs, antihistamines, hypnotics, lithium, opioid analgesics, NSAIDs and selective serontonin reuptake inhibitors (SSRLs) have all been found to impact on incontinence (Wagg and Malone-Lee, 1998).

Freda's incontinence was assessed as being urge incontinence due to reduced mobility and her care plan updated to include more sessions with the physiotherapy team. The multi disciplinary team concluded that although Freda was still in pain she needed to become more independent which in turn would strengthen her and contribute to reducing the pain in her back. Freda was not included in the decision process at this stage as she was noted to complain of increasing pain when she knew movement was required e.g. washing, and openly objected stating that first her pain needed to be addressed. Staff did talk with Freda about mobility and how it will help her in the long run but Freda was distrusting and believed movement would only make things worse. It was felt that Freda would become non compliant if she knew in advance of the recommended increase in physiotherapy sessions, instead the nursing staff would get her to comply by saying things like the bed needed to be changed so she needed to sit out in the chair then the physiotherapist was able to prompt her into attendance "since she was already up".

Becoming incontinent affects lives, continence is paramount in retaining dignity (Turner, 1999). Incontinence is embarrassing, undignified and unpleasant, quality of life is impaired (Geriatric

Medicine, 2009). Approximately sixteen percent of the population are known to have a bladder problem (Office for National Statistic, 2007). Noctural polyuria is when more than 35% of the total urine production occurs during sleep. Having to wake one or more times at night to void called nocturia causes sleep deprivation and can impair cognitive performance during the day and can lead to depression (Turner, 1999). Incontinence can lead to psychological stress due to its unpredictability and odour. Isolation, anxiety and depression can be attributed to incontinence problems (Earthy, 2009). Hygiene can become compromised and lead to skin breakdown. Some urinary tract infections are as a result of incontinence (Earthy, 2009). Having to alter the way you dress to accommodate incontinence can cause problems with individual sexuality and not being able to express your personality through your normal dress sense (NICE, 2006) (Turner, 1999). A large percentage of admission into a healthcare setting is attributed to incontinence (Turner, 1999).

Freda's incontinence was affecting her mood making her more depressed but it was also noted that the more immobile she became due to pain the less she wanted to move which in turn led to increasing her immobility and incontinence. Freda's care plan included maintenance of her personal hygiene by giving assistance and encouraging independence as much as possible and her care plan was updated to include a referral to the "pain team". Freda was informed that the pain team had been asked to review her and she was happy for this to happen. These measures were part of the process to address Freda's incontinence.

People having to live with incontinence, whether for a few days or as an ongoing problem, need reassurance and comfort to retain their self respect. "Maintaining a normal toileting pattern, in a sitting position and in a private space, contributes to improved self esteem and dignity" (Earthy, 2009). It is important to give positive feedback when patients are continent and to prompt voiding as this helps patients to retain their self esteem (NICE, 2006). Good hygiene practices are also paramount to prevent secondary health issues such as skin break down.

Many treatments are available for incontinence depending on its cause. First line treatment is pelvic floor muscle training; carrying out thirty two pelvic contractions per day for at least three months has been shown to benefit (NICE, 2006). Pelvic floor muscle training is recommended to pregnant women in their first pregnancy as a preventative measure against future bladder problems.

Bladder training comprises of muscle strengthening exercises, gradual increase of urination delay, scheduled toileting and keeping of a diary to review effectiveness of the training. Bladder training typically lasts three to twelve weeks.

Drugs such as Oxybutynin an anticholinergic which reduces nerve transmission helps reduce frequency and urgency of passing urine in unstable bladder and with detrusor muscle instability, cognitive impairment in older people has been associated with this drug (Katz, 1998). The health care professionals did not feel drugs or pelvic floor exercises were needed in Freda's case.

Surgical interventions include colposuspension for prolapsed of the vaginal wall, this is when upper vaginal wall is fixed to the anterior abdominal wall. Autologous rectus facial sling to treat stress incontinence is when a graft is made using the rectus muscle to make a sling that holds the bladder neck in place. Another surgical procedure is augmentation cystoplast a means of enlarging the capacity of the bladder by using a section of the bowel. None surgical methods of treatment include firming muscles using intramural bulking agents. As Freda's incontinence resulted from reduced mobility only her treatment option was restricted to physiotherapy only.

Lifestyle changes can improve continence such as reducing caffeine education about fluid intake and output (Dowd, 1996) exercise to improve gait, speed and stamina (Van Houten, 2007) and weight loss. For cognitively impaired patients prompted and timed voiding toileting programs have been shown to help.

Freda's incontinence was a by product of her back pain. The incontinence issue could have been treated with more assistance or toileting aids but it was felt in her case that this would lead to dependence (Donaldson, 2000) and that her incontinence should be addressed by review of medication to alleviate the pain causing the immobility and incontinence. Once Freda felt that something was being done for her pain her compliance to other treatments increased. Freda's mobility increased, her pain was eventually controlled and her incontinence cured. Rather than treating the symptoms of incontinence the care plan was able to identify areas of concern that in turn cured the incontinence.

Good practice for continence care includes assessment, bladder training, pelvic floor exercises, medication review, availability of advice and monitoring (Donaldson, 2000). Pads, urinals, toileting aids are not to be used as a treatment and should only be used if not coping pending definite treatment alongside to therapy or as part of long term management after other options have been explored.

Freda's healthcare issues were addressed using a care plan which was intermittently evaluated by the multidisciplinary team and added to as was necessary to incorporate new health issues Freda experienced during her hospital admission. Freda's consent was not always sought along with her preferences/opinions, likes/dislikes taken into consideration whenever an element of care was being considered. The care plan helped to identify areas that required attention and those that had been successfully addressed. When care plans are followed and updated it makes evaluation easier and helps to identify areas that need review and those areas that have been addressed successfully.

During this care study I have been able to identify an element of care in this case urinary incontinence. I have researched what urinary incontinence is, its causes, effects and treatment and been able to relate it to a patient and see how with the aid of a care plan and patient participation how the problem was addressed and resolved.

Reference

Abrams, Cardozo, Fall (2002), The standardisation of terminology in lower urinary tract function: report from the Standardisation Sub-committee of the International Continence Society, Neurourology and Urodynamics Vol 21(2) pp 167-178

Chiarellil, Brown, McElduff (1999), Leaking Urine: Prevalence and associated factors in Australian women, Neurourology and Urodynamic Vol 18(6) pp 567-577

Donaldson (2000), Good Practice in Continence Services, Department of Health online: www.doh.gov.uk/continenceservices.htm, (Accessed: 18 September 2009)

Dowd, Campbell, Jones (1996), Fluid intake and urinary incontinence in older community-dwelling women

Earthy (2009), Enhanced continence care, www.LTLMAGAZINE.COM (Accessed: 18th September 2009)

Geriatric Medicine (2009), Urinary continence management in older people, Nursing Older People Continence Essentials Guide

Katz, Sands, Bilker (), Identifications of medications that cause cognitive impairment in older people: the case of oxybutynin chloride, Journal of the American Geriatrics Society Vol 46(1) pp 8-13

National Institute for Health and Clinical Excellence (2006), Urinary incontinence: The management of urinary incontinence in women, NICE Clinical guideline 40

Office for National Statistics (2007), Ageing, www.statistics.gov.uk/cci/nugget.asp:ID=949, (Accessed 18th September 2009)

Thompson (2007), Falls and Incontinence: evaluation of a quality management project, Australian and New Zealand Continence Journal Vol 13(1) pp 18-21

Turner, Foster, Johnson (1999), Occupation Therapy and Physical Dystfunction: Principles, Skills and Practice, London, Churchill Livingstone

Van Houten, Achterberg, Ribble (2007), Urinary incontinence to disabled elderly women: a randomised clinical trial on the effect of training mobility and toileting skills to achieve independent toileting, Gerontology Vol 52(4) pp 205-210

Wagg and Malone-Lee (1998), Urinary incontinence in the elderly, British Journal of Urology Vol 82(1) pp 11-17

Chapter 6

What is Group Working?

Group work is a form of cooperative learning. It should cater for individual differences; develop knowledge, generic skills (e.g. communication skills, collaborative skills, critical thinking skills) and attitudes. Group work is essential in nursing studies as it demonstrates ability to communicate, discuss and co-operate, these skills are invaluable in nursing practice.

Group Project
Summary of individual student input

1. Introduction

The aim of the presentation was to gain a more in-depth understanding of the reliability and validity of four assessment tools in general use, and to discover if research support that they are the current best practice or whether more studies are needed.

2. Aim and objectives (4 to 6) of the group presentation

The focus of our group aims were targeted towards our ability to assess relevant research information, and how to analyse the research we found and compare it to current practice. We formulated views and judgments from the research that we felt would influence future practice.
Secondary to this we aimed to develop our ability to work as a team.

3. Objective's that I individually focused upon

My focus was on the Waterlow assessment tool. The main objective for me was to find out if scores obtained from a completed Waterlow assessment tool is valid by measuring the inter rater reliability.

4. Method's I used to achieve my objectives

In order to achieve my objective I conducted an extensive database search using Cinahl, Medline and British Nursing Index. The database retrieved numerous studies whereby I then had to filter out the most relevant to my need which I found in several specialised journals. I was also advantaged by being on placement in an area that uses the Waterlow everyday so I was able to observe its use and compare what I witnessed to what I read.

5. **The key findings from my objectiv'e supported with references.**

The main finding from my research was that inter rater reliability for the Waterlow is not very good according to the studies I reviewed, with the main reason being that it is used without the user knowing how it was originally intended to be used. This finding cast a shadow of concern as to if appropriate care can be delivered based on the Waterlow use. One study highlighted the fact that nurse clinical judgement had an acceptable level of reliability supporting that best practice is being carried out using the Waterlow as an aid and not a diagnostic tool. The Waterlow appears to be used today to justify spending by means by audit. (Gould, Kelly, Goldstone, Gammon (2001), Gould, Goldstone, Gammon, Kelly, Maidwell (2002), Kelly, (2005), Royal College of Nursing (2001).

6. **Key findings of the group (summary) supported with references**

- There is no evidence to suggest that the introduction of MEWS contribute to improved patient outcomes McGaughey, et al, (2009), Subbe, et al, (2003).
- The MUST has been proved to be valid and reliable. If weight and height become an issue then other subjective criteria can be used, especially when patients have fractures, are at risk of falls, a stooping patient, confused patients, unconscious patients or non-compliant patients (Green and Watson, 2005).
- Waterlow is used to make important costly clinical decisions. Study highlights that clinical judgement should not be outweighed by the outcome of a risk assessment score (The European Pressure Ulcer Advisory Panel, 1998).
- Experienced nurses can use the GCS with high levels of reliability and accuracy. Practitioners with limited training and experience can use the GCS with high levels of reliability but the accuracy of their ratings is suspect

and they do less well in scoring (Rowley and Fielding, 1991).

7. Selected references (8 to 10) that support your input into the presentation

Brick, Stephens (2007), Pressure Ulcer Risk Assessment and Prevention: Report of a national audit pilot project, Available at: http://www.rcn.rg.uk/_data/assets/word_ doc/006/109842/pressure_ulcer_audit_pilot _project.doc (Accessed 17th April 2010)

Edwards (1994), The rationale for the use of risk calculators in pressure sore prevention, and the evidence of the reliability and validity of published scales, Journal of Advanced Nursing Vol 20(2) pp 288-296 EBSCO host [Online], Available at: http://0-web.ebscohost.com.brum.beds.ac.uk/ehost/ pdfviewer/pdfviewer?vid=3andhid-15andsid=c0e644cf-2db7-4899-b443-173be04d1134%40sessinmgr10 (Accessed 1st May 2010)

European Pressure Ulcer Advisory Panel (1998). Pressure Ulcer Prevention and Treatment Guidelines. Oxford, EPUAP

Gould, Kelly, Goldstone, Gammon (2001), Examining the validity of pressure ulcer risk assessment scales: developing and using illustrated patient simulations to collect the data, Joural of Clinical Nursing Vol 10(5) pp 697-706 EBSCO host [Online], Available at: http://0-ejscontent.ebsco.com.brum.beds.ac.uk/ContentServer.aspx?target=http%3A%2F%2Fwww3%2Einterscience%2Ewiley%2Ecom%2Fresolve%2Fresolve%2Fdoi%2Fpdf%3FDOI%3D10%2E1046%2Fj%2E1365%2D2702%2E2001%2E00525%2Ex (Accessed 1st May 2010)

Gould, Goldstone, Gammon, Kelly, Maidwell (2002), Establishing the validity of pressure ulcer risk assessment scales: a novel approach using illustrated patient scenarios, International Journal of Nursing Studies Vol 39(2) pp 215-228 EBSCO host [Online}, Available at: (Accessed 1st May 2010)

Kelly (2005), Inter-rater reliability and Waterlow's pressure ulcer risk assessment tool, Nursing Standard Vol 19(32) pp 86-92, EBSCO host Cinahl available online at: http://0-web.ebscohost.com.brum.beds.ac.uk/ehost/pdfviewer/pdfviewer?vid=4andhid=8andsid-0ddc41de-fe70-4a99-85f1-c4ce1b00d30a%40sessionmgr10 (Accessed 17th April 2010)

Royal College of Nursing (2001), Clinical Practice Guidelines: Pressure ulcer risk assessment and prevention. Royal College of Nursing, London

Chapter 7

What is a Learning Contract?

A learning contract is one method of implementing the concepts of self-directed learning. Goals and Objectives: The overall goal of the learning contract is to allow the student to take responsibility for his/her own learning. A learning need is the gap between where you are and where you want to be.

Learning Contract

Pressure Sore Identification and Prevention

In this Learning Contract I have chosen to explore how best to identify pressure sores and promote health by learning how to prevent pressure sores forming or exacerbating existing sores. This learning outcome relates to Unit learning outcome number five. I have chosen pressure sores as they are "chronic, debilitating wounds, which continue to be significant and challenging clinical problems" (Brick and Stephens 2007), and, since pressure sores are reported across all health care settings, affect all age groups and are "costly in terms of quality of life for those who sustain tissue damage, and in terms of demands on health service resources" (European Pressure Ulcer Advisory Panel, 19998). The Royal College of Nursing (2001) state that, "The human and financial cost of pressure ulcers, together with a variation in practice across the UK, and a growing body of knowledge about effectiveness, have highlighted the need for recommendations for practice". These quotes demonstrate a need to effectively address how they should be managed to maximise cost effectiveness on a finite NHS budget while achieving optimal care, and by virtue that patient compliance is require to achieve this, health promotion can only be achieved with effective communication and information giving the skills required to teach patients self care strategies.

To achieve my learning outcomes I shall be defining what a pressure sore is, explore the use of assessment tools to prevent pressure sores, use evidence based knowledge to demonstrate best practice prevention strategies for pressure sores and reflect on my role in supporting patients' in prevention of pressure sores.

A pressure sore could be classified as a wound which is considered an interruption of the skin on the skin surface or underlying tissues (Alexander, 2002). The European Pressure Ulcer Advisory Panel (EPUPAP, 1998) describes a pressure sore as being "an area of localized damage to the skin and underlying tissue caused by pressure, shear, friction and or a combination of these. Pressure sores are then sub categorised into four stages based on what tissue layers are affected and the extent of that damage. Stage one is non blanching erythema over unbroken skin usually over a bony area like the elbow or heel. Stage two is partial thickness loss over intact or broken skin sero-sanginous filled or blister, this stage of sore will have a red wound bed and be absent of slough. Stage three is full thickness skin loss, under lying tendons and muscle will not show but subcutaneous fat may be visible. At this stage the under lying tendons and muscle are till protected by a strong fibrous layer, depth of this stage may be hard to gauge. Stage four is full thickness tissue loss muscle, tendon and or bone exposed with slough present. (EPUPAP, 1998)

As stated above pressure sores can result from pressure, shear and friction or in combination. Immobility is a contributing factor when looking at sores as a result of pressure. Immobility reduces the circulatory effectiveness due to a lower demand being made on the heart for oxygen transportation around the body. When pressure is introduced the circulation is vulnerable to inadequate supply and then has the potential to cause cells to die from lack of oxygen and the start of a pressure sore can follow. Immobility is often made worse in the elderly by lack of confidence due to falls resulting in reluctance to move. Urgency incontinence can also lead to falls and subsequent drop in confidence leading to immobility. It is easy to see from this that when promoting mobility it may be a case of promoting continence that is the issue or that a patient's confidence needs to be restored with rehabilitation.

Shear and friction are other known causes of pressure sores. Poor moving and handling techniques used can cause the skin to break, the movement/force shears off skin leaving a wound which can be great or mall in size. Skin friction results from drag movement and can lead to skin damage. It maybe carers are using inappropriate moving and handling techniques or that a patient is. Both carers and patients need educating on how to avoid skin damage through inappropriate movement. Patients with orthopaedic problems need rehabilitation to regain strength and range of movement that while compromised increases the risk of pressure sore development.

While patients are in hospital it is important from a patient safety point of view to employ strategies that will help prevent pressure sore development and not exacerbate existing sores. Assessment tools are one way of attempting to predict if a patient is at risk of developing a pressure sore. Many studies have been carried out to analyse if risk assessment scales are valid and reliable. A study by Kelly (2005) discovered that nurses scored differently on same patient scenarios when using a risk assessment scale. The difference was mainly due to users of the risk assessment scale not understanding how the scale was intended to be used. No study has been carried out to date that has revisited this study to find out if user education on the risk assessment scales use would improve the inter-rater reliability. An as yet unproven area of research of pressure sore prevention is the effectiveness of nursing intervention or equipment use which due to ethics cannot be fully investigated. The ethical dilemmas limiting research means that assess meant tools can only safely be used in conjunction with clinical expertise as an aid and not as a diagnoses tool. Two other studies by Gould (2001) and Gould

(2002) attempted to validate several pressure sore risk assessment scales against the congruent between clinical nurse and clinical nurse specialists (tissue viability nurse). A pilot study confirmed that the study design was appropriate and various testing procedures found the study methodology suitable. This study demonstrated that results from using risk assessment scales were not influenced by nursing experience or social background and that nursing staff were able to correctly risk assess 82% of the time using a visual analogue scale and 63% using risk assessment scales. The visual analogue scale results demonstrated clearly that risk assessment scales used alongside clinical judgement is effective.

Prevention strategies for prevention of pressure sore development used in National Health Service (NHS) settings include pressure mattress use and turning regime programs. A study published in two thousand and four attempted to measure the effect of a turning program aimed at reducing incidence of pressure sores. It was acknowledged in the study that good skin maintenance kept well moisturised, dry and clean together with good incontinence management and regular turning/re-positioning of patients reduced pressure sore incidence. The reduction in pressure sore incidence was acknowledged in part as contributing to reducing hospital stay and referrals for associated problems such as deep vein thrombosis, emboli and pneumonia arising from reduced mobility. It was also acknowledged that good moving and handling of patients also helped reduced incidence and musculoskeletal injuries to staff. Another finding of the study was reduced nonsocomial infection and incidence of C difficile again related to reduced mobility. (Hobbs 2004).

Pressure relieving mattresses are regularly used in NHS settings. Approximately forty randomised control trials have been carried out on pressure relieving mattresses with most being discredited due to poor methodological faults. Evidence for pressure relieving mattresses comes mostly from testing using dummies with pressure sensors placed on them. This method clearly shows that pressure can be relieved with various mattress types but fails to take into account variables such as nutritional status, body mass index and disease or co morbidities, and uses an average accepted capillary occlusion measurement. It was also noted in studies that effective pressure relief should not be limited to just the bed; chairs should be equipped with a pressure relieving cushion. It does not end here though as unless the chair is customised for the patient bad posture will ensue and therefore make the pressure relieving cushion ineffective. Chairs need to be the right height and width to allow for good posture and adequate pressure relief. (Russel 2001).

As a student nurse I am responsible for my own learning which I have achieved by observing current practice and reading around any given subject in order to be able to deliver safe and effective care which incorporates risk assessment in prevention of illness. Being able to measure the potential harmful effects that may occur if patients are involved with activities, such as reduced mobility, or inappropriate methods of transferring causing friction are equally important (Henderson 1996). The National Institute for Clinical Excellence (NICE) state that a range of parameters should be assessed both base line and regularly thereafter by a first level nurse to help identify risk status of an individual, so knowledge of assessment tools and their reliability and validity is paramount (NICE, 2005). The Royal College of Nursing state that nurses' need to develop their role as a health promoter and educator (RCN, 1989), (DoH, 1989), (Cooper, 2001). By researching risk assessment tools, reading about pressure sore prevention, incidence and formation I have been able to promote good health and preventative strategies while delivering nursing care. I have also learned about the importance of the National Patient Safety Agency (NPSA) a reporting body who specialise in increasing patient safety by analysing incidence of pressure sores. It is written that ten percent of patients admitted into a NHS hospitals experience a safety incident and that about half of these are thought to have been preventable. Seventy two thousand HNS setting incidents contribute to patient death annually (Vincent, 2001). The NPSA describe a patient safety incident as

"Any unintended or unexpected incident which could have or did lead to harm for one or more patient receiving NHS funded care" (NPSA, 2010).

Failure to communicate aspects of patient care and treatment and medical errors are considered safety incidents. The NPSA covers the entire UK's health service and by informing, supporting and influencing people aim to improve safe patient care by reducing risks within the healthcare setting.

In practice I have found that pressure relieving equipment is being used after assessment using a risk assessment scale and combining the result with clinical judgement. Annual moving and handling training keeps staff updated on current best practice, for instance it has recently been found that turning a patient onto their side using a sliding sheet should be carried out using the sliding sheet to position the patient on the bed and then using the log roll, previously it was taught that a combination of pulling the sliding sheet outward and upward would turn the patient safely but risked injury to the turners. An area of concern for me has been the incorrect use of risk assessment scales. I have found that health care professionals are knowledgeable on risk factors for pressure sores and about preventative strategies but not so knowledgeable on how the risk assessment scale in use was intended to be used. This deficit in knowledge is in part countered by clinical judgement.

As a student nurse nearing qualification I feel that I have a duty to inform colleagues about recent research findings regarding pressure relieving products, moving techniques and to question methods used. By doing this I am equipping others with current best practice evidence based, and by questioning methods being used I am ensuring that I am performing tasks with rationale that can be backed up knowing that patients are receiving adequate, safe nursing care.

References

Alexander M (2002), Nursing Practice, Hospital and Home. The adult. (2nd ed). Edinburgh: Churchill Livingstone

Cooper J (2201), A student nurse's learning in a leg ulcer outpatient department, Clinical Practice Vol 12(2) pp 150-161

DoH (1989) A Strategy for Nursing. A Report of the Steering Committee. DoH Nursing Division, London

European Pressure Ulcer Advisory Panel (1998), Pressure Ulcer Treatment Guidelines. Available at: http://www.epuap.org/gltreatment.html (Accessed 15 August 2010)

Gould D, Kelly D, Goldstone L, Gammon J (2001), Examining the validity of pressure ulcer risk assessment scales: developing and using illustrated patient simulations to collect the data, Journal of Clinical Nursing Vol 10(5) pp 697-706 EBSCO host {online}, Available at: http://0-ejscontentebsco.com.brum.beds.ac.uk/ContentS erver.aspx?target=http%3A%2F%2Fwww3%2Ei nterscience%2Ewiley%2Ecom%2Fresolve%2Fdoi %2Fpdf%3D10%2E1046%2Fj%2E1365%3D2702% 2E2001%2E00525%2Ex (Accessed 1st May 2010)

Gould D, Goldstone, Gammon J, Kelly D, Maidwell A (2002), Establishing the validity of pressure ulcer risk assessment scales: a novel approach using illustrated patient scenarios, International Journal of Nursing Studies Vol 39(2) pp 215-228

Henderson V (1996), The nature of Nursing Macmillan Publishing New York

Hobbs B (2004), Reducing the incidence of pressure ulcers: Implementation of a Turn-Team Nursing Program, Journal of Gerontological Nursing Vol 17(3) pp 46-51

Kelly J (2005), Inter-rater reliability and Waterlow's pressure ulcer risk assessment tool, Nursing Standard Vol 19(32) pp 86-92, EBSCO host Cinahl available online at: http://0-web.ebscohost.com.brum.beds.ac.uk/chost/pdf viewer/pdfviewer?vid=4andhid=8andsid=0ddc 41de-fe70-4a99-85fl-c4ce1b00d30a%40sessionmgr10 (Accessed 17th April 2010)

NICE (2205), The Management of pressure Ulcers in Primary and Secondary Care, NICE, London

RCN (1989) Into the Nineties: Promoting Professional Excellence. RCN, London

Royal College of Nursing (2001), Clinical Practice Guidelines: Pressure ulcer risk assessment and prevention. Royal College of Nursing. London

Russell L (2001), Overview of research to investigate pressure-relieving surfaces, British Journal of Nursing Vol 10(21) pp 1421-1426

Vincent C, Neale G and Woloshynowych M (2001) Adverse events in British hospitals: preliminary retrospective record review. British Medical Journal Vol 322(7285), pp 517-519

Chapter 8

What is a Care Study?

For this the student is required to identify a nursing problem for the study, formulate a nursing diagnosis and plan of care using research and reflection on the patient perspective.

Patient centred care in chronic/long term conditions
Case Study

In this case study I will first identify my chosen patient anonymously and the chronic condition(s) that this patient has. My study will include a description about the chronic health condition(s) my patient has experienced along with some of the life changing factors that have arose as a result. Due to the number of factors connected with these types of health conditions I will only be concentrating on one being; pharmacological effects of the drugs on the body and a little on the psychological impact of these conditions and how these have impacted on my patient's experience.

My chosen patient is a thirty five year old Afro Caribbean male who I shall call Mike. Mike worked full time in a busy restaurant as an experienced qualified chef who lives with his girlfriend. Mike is adopted and has no children of his own.

Mikes medical notes show that in 2004 he failed to attend a follow up appointment for suspected mitral murmur. Nothing further is entered into the notes until March 2008 when Mike presented in Accident and Emergency with an Achilles tendon injury caused while playing football. Non steroidal anti inflammatory drugs were prescribed to last for a month and sick not given with duration of seven days.

Later in year Mike attended at his general practitioners (GP) surgery complaining of shortness of breath and was diagnosed as being asthmatic. Within a few days Mike presented at Accident and Emergency (A and E) complaining of shortness of breath and was found to have an enlarged heart. Mike was sent home to await an appointment with a specialist. Less than a month later Mike presented again in accident and emergency with a history of shortness of breath progressing over a period of six weeks, intermittent palpitations, orthopnoea (unable to sleep lying down), PND and an episode of diarrhoea and vomiting a few weeks prior to his visit to his GP. On assessment it was noted that Mike had ankle swelling, elevated Troponin levels, renal impairment but with normal size kidneys and so was admitted for further assessment.

Clinical tests showed a mural thrombus in the left ventricle with an ejection of less than 14%, very severe dilated cardiomyopathy with a hugely dilated left ventricle and dilated right ventricle with very poor biventricular function, no myocarditis or cardiomyopathy was identified. The diagnosis was recorded as dilated cardiomyopathy in December 2008 after trips to hospitals in Milton Keynes, Oxford and Harefield.

Dilated cardiomyopathy (DCM) accounts for approximately 15% of all types of heart failures and is the leading reason for heart transplantation (NICE, 2003). DCM is diagnosed when dilation of the left ventricular with systolic dysfunction is found not to be caused by hypertension or valve disease. The increase in the chamber size increases the load on the heart and often presents with right ventricular dilation and dysfunction (Elliot et al, 2008). DCM is more common in African American people (Bruce, 2005) and is often found to be an inherited condition (Walker, 2008), in Mike's case due to being adopted it was impossible to prove or disprove whether his condition came about through a faulty inherited gene or caused by a virus. Mike's presenting symptoms at A and E were in line with symptoms associated with DCM being dyspnoea, orthopnoea, palpitations, unexplained syncope (Walker, 2008), and, ejection fraction of less than 45% (Elliot et al, 2000). DMC is a disabling condition has a poor prognosis with the only treatment being heart transplantation. Medication is used to treat the symptoms before hear transplantation (Walker, 2008).

The realisation of knowing that you need a heart transplant is very traumatic for the person concerned, in this case Mike, understandably brings about fear as there is an awareness that your life is under constant and immediate threat (Spilsbury, 2008). Physical and psychological processes continue before surgery until years after requiring ongoing assessment and treatment (Dressler, 1993). Psychological distress is known to remain for several years after heart transplantation (Reyes et al, 2003). Post operatively over one to five years emotional ell being deteriorates significantly (Bunzel et al, 1999). Psychological and physiological rejection of a heart is sometimes associated (Rauch and Kneen, 1989) so it is important for Mike to adjust and come to terms with his condition. Mike had lots to take in not just the physical implication of his condition. Mikes biggest concern was whether he would be able to continue working. The severity of Mike's condition became critical and necessitated Mike having to have an operation to fit an artificial pump to take over the work of the left side of his heart. The operation was successful. It was hoped that the pump would allow the right side of his heart to recover but this unfortunately did not happen and Mike had to endure another operation to fit a second pump. During this second operation Mike had a stroke which was quickly identified and thus a treatment regime was untaken quickly to reduce its effects.

Approximately 11% of deaths in the UK are from stroke, most people survive the first stroke. 110,000 people per annum have a stroke and 20,000 a TIA, nearly one million people are living with the after effects of stroke at any one time with around £7 billion per annum being spent annually on treatments with nearly half of this born directly by the NHS (NICE, 2008). NICE guidelines state that stroke is both treatable and preventable, identification of people at higher risk of stroke allows for better intervention practice being used to minimise the risk of stroke occurring or reoccurring. Evidence indicated that first treatment greatly improves outcome and that a key part of care is to prevent exacerbating brain damage caused by stroke by maintenance of cerebral blood flow and oxygenation. As Mike's stroke was identified almost immediately he was able to receive care and therapy in line with NICE guideline 68. As a nurse you are expected to know of the guideline and what the recommendation are for nursing someone with a particular ailment and be able to implement this into the patient care plan. The guidelines "are recommendations about the treatment and care of people with specific diseases and conditions in the NHS in England and Wales" (NICE, 2008).

The combination of stroke and heart failure meant Mike has to take a variety of medications to reduce his symptoms of heart failure and help prevent re-occurrence of stroke. Some of the medications prescribed to Mike their use and implications are discussed below.

Furosemide is a loop diuretic used for pulmonary oedema and heart failure usually left ventricular failure it reduces symptoms of shortness of breath. Furosemide works by preventing re-absorption from the ascending limb of the loop of henle in the renal tubal by preventing transportation of sodium chloride out of the distal tubal into the interstitial tissues. By increasing the urinary output and reducing the plasma volume the venous return is lowered and pre load on the cardiac muscle reduced Furosemide acts within one hour of taking and completes within 6 hours so it best given during the day preferably morning to prevent nocturia. The reduced workload on the hear can cause hypotension and hypokalaemia (muscle weakness) continued monitoring is advisable until the patient is accustomed to the drug therapy (BMA, 2007, BNF 2008 and Hopkins, 2007). As Mike is aware of exercising increasing his hearts workload the knowledge that this loop diuretic will increase urinary output equalling more trips to the toilet can be a stressing factor. Mike needs to understand how this medication works and its benefits as this information helps patients to understand the need to take the drug and lead to better compliance and thus better health outcome.

Warfarin is prescribed to prevent venous thrombosis and pulmonary embolism to treat cerebral ischemia and to prevent formation of clots; this is achieved by maintaining an INR value of between two and three. INR stands for International normalised ratio (prothrombin time) which is time that it takes for your blood to clot (platelet forming). Warfarin works by blocking the antagonists vitamin K. 3mg is recommended for dilated cardiomyopathy and mural thrombus in line with Mikes prescribed dose. A nursing point to remember is that this drug should be taken at the same time every day to avoid changes in the blood level of warfarin. As this drug prevents/reduces clotting time haemorrhage is always a risk and bleeding gums and erythrocytes in urine should be observed as a warning sign of possible overdose (BMA, 2007, BNF, 2008 and Hopkins 2007). Mike needs to be educated on his medication so that he can self medicate once he returns home, a huge responsibility.

Amiodarone is used to correct arrhythmias it is a calcium channel blocker which reduces contraction strength by extending the refractory period of the contractile fibres of both atria and ventricles. The refractory period is when calcium ions move into the cell and at that stage the muscle cells will not respond to further stimulation. The cardiac cycle is dependent on the movement of sodium, potassium and calcium ions in and out of the heart muscle; interference of calcium here slows the nerve response. As this is an iodine containing drug problems with thyroid function can occur, Amiodarone also increases the response to Warfarin so this has to be adjusted accordingly. Initial response to Amiodarone is slow and hypotension needs to be monitored (BMA, 2007, BNF, 2008 and Hopkins 2007). Amiodarone should only be prescribed after specialist consultation (NICE, 2003). Knowing that all drugs can have side effects and possibly cause secondary health problems can be an additional worry and highlights the need for patient education to increase compliance with treatment.

Bisoprolol is a beta blocking agent that protects the heart from excessive stimulation physical or emotional stress. Beta blockers are usually used with ace inhibitors and a diuretic to treat hypertension. Beta blockers interrupt the transmission of stimuli through beta receptors, they block actions which originate in the adrenal glands and act mainly on beta I receptors located mainly in the heart muscle. By slowing the heart rate and reducing the force of the heart beat the workload on the cardiac muscle is reduced. The side effects of this therapy are that it can reduce the capacity for exercise, reduce circulation which can lead to impotence (BMA 2007, BNF 2008 and Hopkins 2007). As an active thirty five year old male coming to terms with reduced physical capability and its indirect effects such as not being able to work and support your family can lower your self esteem.

The chronic conditions that Mike now has to live with means he has to deal with many life changing factors. Factors include a changing body image as Mike now has to wear a back pack all the time apart from when he is sleeping; the backpack holds the batteries necessary for Mike's artificial pumps to keep working. This in itself is quite challenging physically and emotionally as firstly the batteries are heavy and secondly you have the burden of having to remember to change and charge them, sleeping in could cost Mike his life! As a chef Mike likes to dine out but now has to consider where he can go without his backpack looking out of place eg: wearing a backpack with a suit will naturally draw attention. The aforementioned gives rise to social isolation but also due to physical weakness arising from the stroke making even a short trip to the shops an ordeal worrying whether there will be somewhere he can sit down for a rest, awareness of a crowd being unaware of his condition and pushing past can be emotionally distressing.

Psychologically Mike has to come to terms with his reduced weakness resulting in his inability to work and continue to be the main bread winner, needing equipment to aid his independence in carrying out daily tasks such as washing and eating. Mike's frail body means he is more fearful not just of the immediate threat his failed heart poses but fear of common illness such as flu. Sexual health is another issue studies have shown that erectile dysfunction is seen in men with heart disease or men receiving treatment for hear failure/disease (Dunn et al, 1999). It is also known that Beta blocker reduce libido (Weiss, 1991) and men experience ejaculatory problems (Hale and Strassberg, 1990). Mike is a thirty five year old male so his sexual health is of concern to him and at least one of the drugs he is taking is known to cause impotence. Breathing problems, pain in your chest and an irregular heartbeat during sexual intercourse have revealed in studies to make people think of their bodies as fragile and in turn leads to negative thinking of their bodies and lead to problems with physical and sexual activities as a fear has been generated of provoking the disease this fear is not supported by evidence which shows that virtually no difference is found between people living with heart failure/disease or the general population. It seems that the psychological factors seems more of a problem than any medical problem (Traeen et al, 2007) (Verplanken et al, 2005) (Bernardo, 2001).

National guidelines such as those published by NICE have greatly improved quality of life for some people by identifying best practise based on current evidence but these remain subjective to those following them who have to call upon their own clinical experience and knowledge of health/illness and awareness of guidelines and how to best implement them in their care plans.

In conclusion my study has highlighted some of the problems that chronic conditions can have on patients impacting on their lives physically and psychologically. My study has show how medication can alleviate symptoms and how it can affect sexuality, cure effect our psychological well being and illness affect our social standing.

Reference

Bernardo (2001), The measurement of psychological androgyny, Journal of Consulting and Clinical Psychology Vol 442 pp 155-162

BMA (2007), Henry (editor) Concise Guide To Medicines And Drugs, London, Dorling Kindersley

BNF (2008), British National Formulary, London, BMJ Group and RPS Publishing

Bruce (2005), Getting to the heart of cardiomyopathies, Nursing Vol 35(8) pp 44-47

Bunzel, Laederach-Hofmann (1999), Long-term effect of heart transplantation: The gap between physical performance and emotion well-being, Scandinabian Journal of Rehabilitation Medicine Vol 31(4) pp 214-222

Dictionary.com (no date), Dictionary.com, [online] Available at: http://dictionary.reference.com/browse/happiness, (Accessed 24th June 2009)

Dressler (1993), Transplantation in end-stage hear failure, Critical Care Nursing Clinics of North America Vol 3 pp 635-647

Dunn, Droft, Hacken (1999), Sexual problems: A study of the prevalence and need for health care in the general population, Family Practise Vol 15 pp 519-524

Elliot, Anderson, Arbuttini, (2000), Diagnosis and management of dilated cardiomyopath, Heart Vol 84 pp 106-112

Elliot, Anderson, Arbuttini (2008), Classification of the cardiomyopathies: A position statement from the European Society of Cardiology working group on myocardial and pericardial disease, Eur Heart vol 29 pp 270-276

English Dictionary (2002), Pocket English Dictionary, London, Dorling Kindersley

Hallstrom, Strassebery (1990), Changes in women's sexual desire in middle life: The longitudinal study of women in Gothenbury, Archives of Sexual Behaviour Vol 20 pp 171-186

Hopkins (2007), Drugs and Pharmacology for Nurses, London, Chruchill Livingstone

National Collaborating Centre for Chronic Conditions (2003), Chronic heart failure Management of chronic heart failure in adults in primary and secondary care, NICE Clinical Guideline 5

National Collaborating Centre for Chronic Conditions (2008), Stroke Diagnosis and initial management of acute stroke and transient ischemic attack (TIA), NICE Clinical guideline 68

Rauch, Kneen (1989), Accepting the gift of life: Heart transplant recipients postoperative adaptive tasks, Social Work and Health Care Vol 14 pp 47-59

Reyes, Evangelista, Doering, Dracup, Cesario, Kobashigawa (2003), Physical and psychological attributes of fatigue in female heart transplant recipients, The Journal of Heart and Lung Transplantation Vol 23(5) pp 614-619

Spilsbury (2008), Middle-aged people with chronic heart failure experienced the frustration of living with an unpredictable and failing body, Journal of Evidence Based Nursing Vol 11(1) pp 32-34

Traeen, Olsen (2007), Sexual dysfunction and sexual well-being in people with heart disease, Sexual and Relationship Therapy Vol 22(2) pp 193-208

Verplanken (2006), Beyond frequency: Habit as a mental construct, British Journal of Social Psychology Vol

Verplanken, Friborg, Wang, Trafimow, Wolf (2005), Negative self-thinking as dysfunctional habit: A Process measure Vol

Walker (2008), An introduction to dilated cardiomyopathy, British Journal of Cardiac Nursing Vol 3(11) pp 506-510

Weiss (1991), Effects of antihypertensive agents on sexual function, American Family Physician Vol 44 pp 2075 -2082

Chapter 9

What is Group Working?

Group work is a form of cooperative learning. It should cater for individual differences; develop knowledge, generic skills (e.g. communication skills, collaborative skills, critical thinking skills) and attitudes. Group work is essential in nursing studies as it demonstrates ability to communicate, discuss and co-operate, these skills are invaluable in nursing practice.

Group Presentation
An Account

As part of my ongoing learning I was required to put together a presentation that would demonstrate my ability to analyse existing evidence for current nursing practice. The main purpose of this was to formulate views and judgments that may affect the development of future nursing practice. To discourage bias this project was carried out within a group. The subject was left open for the group to decide.

My group consisted of three other nursing students.

Initially we discussed as a group what subject areas we felt would be relevant. At this stage there was no structure to our group and ideas were thrown in randomly without much thought being put into how the various subjects could be divided between the group members in a logical sequence that would follow on from each other to formulate the presentation. Many hours of potential progress were lost at this stage. Eventually I came up with the idea of discussing assessment tools and their credibility. This subject appeared to be very simple and indeed the rest of the group agreed. From this point on I seemed to have taken on the role of unelected leader with the other group members looking to me for structure. As my background is in management I was more than happy to take on this role. Now that the subject was decided we agreed to go away and do some generalised research of the literature and then meet up to discuss our findings and formulate a plan of action.

For me being chairman was beneficial as I am someone who needs structure to work at my best. At our meeting every one shared with the group their findings, their preference as to which assessment tool they would like to research and ideas on what our group aims should be. It became apparent that one of the group members was struggling to find material so we all agreed to go away and research material for our group member and arranged a future date to meet again to finalise our plan. Myself and another group member arranged to meet with a librarian to get advice on how to refine our research approach. This information proved to be invaluable, we were shown databases that none of us had any knowledge of and learned how to refine our search skills.

Before our next meeting I had encounters with students from a different group to ours who were having difficulty with the tasks set within their own group. I was told in confidence that their own group was not very supportive and that despite their pleas for help from their colleagues they were told it is their problem and that they should sort it out as they all had their own tasks to work on. The main issue was that these particular individuals were having difficulty finding relevant literature to research. I was disappointed to hear about their problems as I thought that as a cohort we were generally very supportive of one another. The knowledge my colleague and I had acquired from the librarian we shared with our other group members and extended this outside to all members of the other groups. Our theory was that one day we will be working with people with whom we may require to support us and encourage our own continued learning. We understood that by sharing knowledge and experience we increase our own learning. I also made time to sit with my fellow colleagues and helped them to source relevant information. The result of our intervention was that one of the other group members wanted to leave the group she was in and join ours. Within my own group we discussed the problems that the other group were having and agreed that although it was unfortunate we were unable to help as we believed that part of the group project involved working as a team and that that meant solving any issues that may arise along the way. We discussed our thoughts with the other group member who agreed with our reasoning.

At this point of our preparation we all started placements. We were all based in different locations, two group members were doing community placements 9am to 6pm and two were doing ward shift work. To complicate things further two members of the group lived outside of the area. All group members had personal commitments with work obligations and children. At our next meeting I gave everyone an analytical template to work by. We confirmed our individual choice of subject and as a group decided on our group aims for the presentation. It was decided that we would not meet for a few weeks so that we had time to complete our individual parts of the presentation.

Finally three out of the four members of our group had completed the individual parts of the presentation so we decided to meet to put it all together. One of the four members was constantly unavailable, never responding to phone calls, text messages or emails. As time was running out the remaining three members decided to meet and put the presentation together without the fourth member. Since I was chairman another group member took on the role of deciding the format for the presentation and jointly we split our group aims (each of us taking one) to be answered. We discussed the un obtain ability of the fourth member and agreed that all we could do was keep trying to contact her and in the mean time carry on with what we could. We met several times after this (without the fourth member) and completed our presentation.

Prior to placement a room had been booked for rehearsal and much to our surprise the fourth member turned up but without their part of the presentation complete. This member asked us to complete it for her, we said no, as we all felt that she was being extremely unfair as we had all had our own personal issues to deal with and had overcome them. We felt that in a real life working situation this individual would probably loss their job due to simply not turning up and not having the courtesy to inform anyone that she wasn't coming or sharing her difficulties which would allow for contingency measures to be put in place and support for her if appropriate. One article I read stated that failure of team members not doing their share or replying on others in patient care can result in reduced nursing care which has its own implications and is after all the main objective. "The purpose of nursing teams is to provide the best possible nursing care for patients" (Castledine, 2010). Another article I read stressed that sharing information and problems is vital for a team (Ashurst, Taylor, 2010). From this I can see how important it is for all group members to be actively involved in order to achieve our common goal.

We did agree to taking her hand written presentation when done and transferring into computer format and integrating it within the main presentation. There was a lot of bitterness between the three members who had completed the work towards the fourth member but this was never expressed to the fourth member as we understood that discord between our team members could result in our main objective not being reached.

Our group met a final time for a rehearsal but this time I was unable to attend due to my own working commitments but I did email a proof read version of the presentation with accompanying notes to them for consideration. Later that day one of the group members phoned me with an update of what had happened and what needed to be tweaked. I arranged to meet with one of the group members the following day to help do the final amendments and we then emailed the other members the final draft of the presentation. We also emailed them with the proposed running order of the presentation and the rational for this.

Reflecting on the whole experience I feel that we achieved what was required a feat in its own right. The good elements of this experience are that we were able to agree on a plan of action and even without the input from one member were still able to complete the task set. We also had our own individual strengths that we recognised and took advantage of, for instance I was chairman, another member was our I.T. specialist and another was good at researching. Again Castledine (2010) stated that "The emphasis of team nursing is on making use of the capabilities of every worker for the good of each patient" in our scenario it was for the good of the presentation. Another major quality of our group was our willingness to help other colleagues and contain negative thoughts so that it didn't affect the progress of the task set. With hind sight I feel that we let our own feelings interfere with the quality of our project. Our focus was temporarily removed from the task set to one of personal gripe towards the member who failed to pull their weight. Had we remained focused on the task set I feel that our grade may have been higher.

I don't really think that we could have completed the task any more efficiently as group work relies on all participants and that in the real world people's personal circumstances will always pose unique individual problems. Once we recognised each other's strengths we were able to exploit these. Each member bar one played a unique role within the group and this I feel gave each member a sense of value which boosts confidence and reflected in the outcome of our work. Equally the outward support that was shown towards the none participating member of our group made her fee valued and supported helping her to achieve her part of the presentation. According to Cioffi, Ferguson (2009), support is an aspect rated highly in one article as beneficial to team work.

If I ever have to carry out a project like this again I would tackle it slight differently. The main difference for me would be to set ground rules and consequences for breaking them. I also feel that this type of working needs to have a structured communication method and that it is important that each member understands their role and what to do if they encounter problems. I naturally assumed a leadership role in this instance but can see that I have a lot to learn as I failed to take responsibility for our team's performance when it came to one member underperforming which is critical to team effectiveness (Tiedeman and Lookinland, 2004). The Nursing and Midwifery Council (2009) states that "You should be aware of, and develop, your ability to communicate effectively within teams". In order for me to improve on my nursing practice I can see that I need to take time out to reflect in order that I can balance my beliefs against evidence.

References

Ashurst and Taylor (2010), Communication, communication, communication, Nursing and Residential Car Vol 12(3) pp 140-142

Castledine (2010), "Team nursing: finding the ideal", British Journal of Nursing Vol 19(13) pp 868-869, EBSCO hot Cinahl [Online] Available at http://0-web.ebscohost.com.brum.beds.ac.uk/ehost/pdfviewer/pdfviewer?vid=11andhid=17andsid=c754549e-96ec-4245-8f0e-e6f90e838322%40sessionmgr14 (Accessed: 28th July 2010)

Cioffi, Ferguson (2009), Team nursing in acute care settings, Contemporary Nurse Vol 33(1) pp 3-12 EBSCO host Cinahl [Online] Available at: http://0-web.ebscohost.com.brum.beds.ac.uk/ehost/pdfviewer/pdfviewer?vid=11andhid=17andsid=c754549e-96ec-4245-8f0e-e6f90e838322%40sessionmgr14 (Accessed: 28th July 2010)

Nursing and Midwifery Council (2009), "Record keeping: Guidance for nurses and midwives"

Available at: http://nmc-uk.org (Accessed 28th July 2010)

Tiedeman and Lookinland (2004), "Traditional models of care delivery: What have we learned?" Journal of Nursing Administration Vol 34(6) pp 291-297

Chapter 10

What is a reflective essay?

A reflective essay is a form of writing that examines and observes the progress of the writer's individual experience. Reflective essays explain and analyze the development of the writer, and discuss future goals.

Group Presentation
Reflective Essay

The fragmented nature of healthcare means that team work is crucial for its success (Salmon D, Jones M, 2001). As part of my own ongoing learning I was required to put together a presentation that would demonstrate ability to analyse existing evidence for current nursing practice as part of a four member student nurse group, enabling the group to formulate views and judgments that may affect the development of future nursing practice. The purpose of this essay is to examine the process of how our group interacted to achieve the end product. Gibbs model of reflection (1998) will be used to break down the experience into six areas; description, feelings, evaluation, analysis, conclusion and action plan. Thorpe (2004) stated that nursing students written reflective journals promote active learning. Reflection is the process of becoming self aware and being able to critic your own actions and behaviour in any given situation (Burns and Bulman, 2000).

DESCRIPTION

Our group was formed in the classroom where we discussed several choices of topic. Brown R (1998) cited by Infed (2010) defines a group as "a group exists when two or more people define themselves as members of it and when its existence is recognized by at least one other". The Collins online dictionary 2010 describes a group as being a number of people or things considered as a unit. As a group we agreed to go off individually and research areas of possible interest for discussion at our next meeting. The topic was jointly agreed and divided into four areas of interest equipping each group member with a unique role. Our group had no structure which was a great frustration to me. At our next meeting I vocalised our need for structure and presented an analytical template for consideration and time line of set targets which was accepted by the group. I was trying to encourage group involvement so that we could collaboratively achieve our common goal. Colbeck et al (2000) states that the term "collaborative learning" is when students "work together as they apply course material to answer questions, solve problems, or create a product" using a variety of instructional practices. As a group we were experiencing the forming stage of Tuckmans's (1995) four stages of group development, the others being storming, norming and performing. Many hours of potential progress were lost at this stage. According to Pearce (2007) time is irreplaceable meaning that success is dependent on effective time management skills.

Our group progressed to Tuckman's (1965) norming stage of group development while individuals within the group went about carrying out their own research in their chosen subject area.

FEELINGS

The "storming" stage of group development came about in two stages, firstly when I tried to bring structure into the group and secondly when one of our group members was failing to adhere to the groups agreed agenda. The group member's non compliance was having an adverse affect on the overall progress of the presentation. Ashurst and Taylor (2010) stated that sharing information and problems is vital for a team. According to Bourner et al (2001) "group-work participation can also be important in promoting the development of time management skills that directly contributes to student autonomy". There was a lot of frustration between the participating group members toward the noncompliant member of the group. As a group we were failing to make use of the capabilities of every worker for the good of our common goal (Castledine, 2010). The reason for our frustration was that we did not know how to deal with the situation.

To overcome this problem we delegated an individual to try and contact the group member concerned. A variety of communication methods were used including text, phone, email and discussion board but without the co-operation of this group member to acknowledge any form of communication we were unable to progress. The Nursing and Midwifery Council (2009) states that "You should be aware of, and develop you ability to communicate effectively within teams".

As the deadline for completion of our presentation was approaching the group member who had been unobtainable came forward and explained her predicament. We discussed the issues raised as a group and agreed upon a plan of action to support our fellow group member and facilitate the completion of our presentation. Coioffi and Ferguson (2009) say that support is an aspect rated highly as beneficial to team work. Our group would have benefited from good leadership in this instance as effective leaders can identify needs and formulate action plans to achieve their goal or in improving a situation (Warren, 2008). Our group by means of this meeting and other previous meetings to discuss progress and feedback had fulfilled Tuckman's (1995) stage of group development "performing". Tuckman later added a fifth stage for the dissolution of a group called adjourning which is when the group reflect and discusses the learning taken place to achieve the group objective, this part of our group development has been achieved by each of us writing a reflective account of our group experience (Tuckman, Jensen, 1977).

EVALUTATION

To make a value judgement Jukes and Vassel (2009) state that this is achieved by asking ourselves what was good and bad about the experience and how the experience made us feel and react. The most positive theme to emerge from this experience was our ability to function as a team and overcome problems with a positive outcome. The experience highlighted my need to be more aware of how team work can enhance learning. Learning and thinking is promoted by encouragement of individuals to participate together (Toofany, 2007). I have also increased my knowledge acquisition through experience in areas of delegation, leadership and due to having to re-submit this assignment improved on my own learning and understanding of self.

The negative aspects were the realisation that despite best efforts my own and that of the other group members personal feelings interfered with best judgement, as although as a group we supported each other we were reluctant to fully support a team member who was struggling as we failed to recognise that this was a team issue and treated it as a personal one effecting only the member concerned. Secondly due to not being able to identify the problems within our group time management was unable to be managed effectively, in contrast this negative aspect has taught me that effective communication helps to facilitate good time management.

ANALYSIS

Each member of our group had their own agenda to complete to facilitate completion of our task but we had no set roles within the group. Our failure to elect a leader with a clear defined role meant that we were not accountable to any one, or in other words had no responsibility individually which is why when a member of our group failed to contribute we were unable to address the problem. Tiederman and Lookinland (2004) states taking responsibility for the team's performance is critical to team effectiveness. I feel that the main reason for this was that we perceived each other of equal status and therefore it was hard to elect a leader, as the word leader in itself suggests someone capable of leading which in contrast could suggest superiority. Had we defined roles it would probably have been easier to appoint members to roles without any personal feelings of impudence.

When the issue arose with one member not fully partaking in the group project I initially along with the other members viewed it as a personal problem unique to that member. Subsequent reading has revealed that "passenger" students are not uncommon and usually associated with relatively long projects or when there are periods of student inactivity (Bourner et al 2001), as we were all on placements for most of this project I can see how this situation was allowed to manifest.

I feel that our completion of the task was due in part to our individual commitment to our chosen subject, Wood (2003) says that giving students a sense of ownership over their learning has shown to increase student performance. In our case choosing our topic proved this as we were more willing to meet in our own time to discuss our individual progress, something that happens much less frequently when we (our cohort) are willing to do when we are all working on the same assignment.

CONCLUSION

Although our group achieved its objective it could have been achieved in a more effective way. As a team we focused on the task set being the presentation completely overlooking group/team work and how it works. Lejk and Wyvill (1996) "propose that by working in a group setting, students achieve competence in tasks directly associated with learning about being effective in teams." Sweeney et al 2008 state that individuals are exposed to potential enhanced higher learning when working in a group.

Had we spent some time researching group effectiveness we could have adopted a better structure to the group. Our group's lack of structure meant we had no clear idea about what each group member role in the group was. Another failing of our group was that we did not define fully any structured communication method or procedure to follow in event of any problems arising, but simply relied on every one complying on an ad hoc basis. Zavertnik et al (2010) said that "development of effective communication in the health care setting should begin in the nursing education program". A study by Roter (2004) showed that communication skill training increased partnership building and problem solving highlighting our/my need to revisit communication skills taught in previous lectures.

ACTION PLAN

If this scenario was to arise again I would want a more structured approach. I feel that it is important that all individuals within the group agree on the aim(s) of the group and what individual roles are. Roles within the group should be defined and agreed so that everyone knows who is responsible for what. Another important aspect would be to formulate a policy to follow when problems arise, on the process of how problems should be addressed and to agree on a communication method.

Now that I have reflected on this experience I feel better apt to cope with team working and challenging situations as this practical experience allowed me to identify deficits in my knowledge base of team working and how to overcome them. Reflecting has also enabled me to apply theory to practice. According to Somerville and Keeling (2004) reflective practice is part of the requirement for nurses constantly to update professional skills. The Nursing and Midwifery Council (2002) state that nurses are responsible for providing care to the best of their ability to patients and their families; this is partly achieved with reflective writing.

References

Ashurst, Taylor (2010), "Communication, communication, communication", Nursing and Residential Care Vol 12(3) pp 140-142

Bourner et al (2001), "First-year Undergraduate Experiences of Group project Work", Assessment and Evaluation in Higher Education Vol 26(1) pp 19-39

Burns and Bulman (2002), Reflective Practice in Nursing 2nd edition, Blackwell Science Limited, Oxford

Castledine (2010), "Team nursing: finding the ideal", British Journal of Nursing Vol 19(13) pp 868-869, EBSCO hot Cinahl [Online] Available at http://0-web.ebscohost.com.brum.beds.ac.uk/ehost/pdf viewer/pdfviewer?vid=11andhid=17andsid=c75 4549e-96ec-4245-8f0e-e6f90e838322%40sessionmgr14 (Accessed: 28th July 2010)

Cioffi, Ferguson (2009), Team nursing in acute care settings, Contemporary Nurse Vol 33(1) pp 3-12 EBSCO host Cinahl [Online] Available at: http://0-web.ebscohost.com.brum.beds.ac.uk/ehost/pdf

viewer/pdfviewer?vid=11andhid=17andsid=c75
4549e-96ec-4245-8f0e-
e6f90e838322%40sessionmgr14 (Accessed: 28th
July 2010)

Colbeck (2000) "Grouping in the dark" Journal
of Higher Education Vol 71(1) pp 60-78
Collins Language.com (2010) "Free Dictionary",
Available at:
http://www.collinslanguage.com/results.aspx?
context=3andreversed=Falseandaction=definean
dhomonym=-1andtext=group, (Accessed 26th
October 2010)

Gibbs (1998) "Learning y Doing: A guide to
teaching and learning methods", Oxford:
Further Education Unit, Oxford Brookes
University

Infed (2010), "What is a group" Available at:
http://www.infed.org/groupwork/what_is_a_
group.html (Accessed 27th October 2010)

Jukes, Vassel (2009), "Delivering a learning
disability education programme in India"
Learning Disability Practice, Vol 12(9) pp 21-25

Lejk, Wyvill (2001), Peer Assessment of
Contributions to a Group Project: A Comparison
of Holistic and Category-based Approaches.

Assessment and Evaluation in Higher
Education, Vol 26(1) pp 61-72.
Nursing and Midwifery Council (2009), "Record
keeping: Guidance for nurses and midwives"
Available at: http://nmc-uk.org (Accessed 28th
July 2010)

Pearce (2007), Ten steps to managing time,
"Nursing Management", Vol 14(1) pp 23-24

Roter, Larson, Shinitzky, Chernoff, Swewint,
Adamo, et al (2004), Use of an innovative video
feedback technique to enhance communication
skills training, Medical Education Vol 38 pp 145-
157

Salmon, Jones, (2001), "Shaping the
interprofessional agenda: a study examining
qualified nurses" perceptions of learning with
others. Nurse Education Today Vol 21(1) pp 18-
25

Somerville and Keeling (2004), "A Practical
approach to promote reflective practice within
nursing." Vol 100(12) pp 42, Available at:
http://www.nursingtimes.net/204502.article,
(Accessed: 26 October 2010)

Sweeney, Weaven and Herington (2008),
"Multicultural Influences on Group Learning: A

Qualitative Higher Education Study",
Assessment and Evaluation in Higher Education
Vol 33(2) pp 119-132

Torpe (2004) "Reflective learning journals: from
concept of practice", Reflective Practice Vol 5(3)
pp 327-343

Tiedeman and Lookinland (2004), "Traditional
models of care delivery: What have we
learned?" Journal of Nursing Administration
Vol 34(6) pp 291-297

Toofany (2007) "Team building and leadership:
the key to recruitment and retention", Nursing
Management Vol 14(1) pp 24-27

Tuckman (1965), "Developmental sequence in
small groups", Psychological bulletin Vol 61(6)
pp 384-399

Tuckman, Jensen (1977) Stages of small group
development revisited. Groups and
Organizatioal Studies, Vol 2(4) pp 419-427
Warren (2008), "Leadership Characteristics", The
Journal of School Nursing Vol 24(3) pp 107-110

Wood (2003) "The Effects of Creating
Psychological Ownership among Students in

Group Project", Journal of Marketing Education Vol 25(3) pp 241-249

Zavertnik, Huff, Munro (2010), "Innovative Approach to Teaching Communication Skills to Nursing Student", Journal of Nursing Education Vol 49(2) pp 65-71

Chapter 11

What is a narrative essay?

A narrative essay firstly outlines a topic based on a clinical situation or event, and describes the aspects of nursing which is going to be explored. The essay should then enable examination and reflection on nursing practice or analyse the situation/event.

Respecting autonomy re right to smoke should healthcare professionals be able to say don't smoke the ethics and moral principles?

The EBL scenario gave an account of George a sixty eight year old male diagnosed with terminal lung cancer being cared for at home who continued to smoke at least twenty cigarettes a day against his family's wishes. The focus of my essay is to identify and explore the ethical dilemma smoking poses for healthcare providers caring for George. I will define autonomy, ethics and moral and then explore their philosophical meaning and their relevance to healthcare.

The principle of self government/autonomy is the individual right of people to self determination. Autonomy is accepted as an unspoken rule in life except when an individual's capacity is compromised preventing them from being able to make informed decisions. Society consensus on personal autonomy has changed over time changing the way treatment is offered to patients away from paternalistic care given by healthcare professionals to care being provided based on the patients locus of control. The question as to whether health outcomes have been compromised as a result of the shift of control from doctor to patient remains unanswered as medical variables are always changing through research and technology and the ethical issues that would arise in formulating a quantitative study would make it difficult to implement.

In the EBL scenario George exercises his autonomy by refusing to quit smoking. The healthcare providers are now left with the ethical dilemma of whether they respect George's autonomous decision knowing the ill effects smoking causes, or whether they take the paternalistic stance of forbidding George from smoking in order to optimise George's health. It is important to understand firstly what ethics means to fully understand the dilemma and ultimately the resolve Ethics in its simplest form are the principles underpinning moral judgement, "a system of morally correct conduct" (English Dictionary, 2002). Correct conduct according to Mill a British philosopher states "the right way to act is to produce the greatest amount of happiness overall" (Mill, 2007). Logically a moral dilemma is a conflict between two moral principles both of which have the capacity for good (Macniven, 19993). Morals are further complicated as they are subjective in that individuals perceive issues/dilemmas based on emotive components through their own personal life experience.

Patient choice through respect for autonomy can conflict with beneficence whereby a patient may choose a treatment or behaviour not in their best interest. Beneficence could be seen as core to medical ethics by definition, as healing is the main purpose of healthcare taking actions to serve the best interest of the patient(s). Non malfeasance or the act of not causing harm to patients is an everyday dilemma healthcare practitioners face as many medicines cause side effects, the rule here is to make sure that the benefits outweigh the risks so non malfeasance often has to be balanced with beneficence. When considering non malfeasance it is important to remember that it is limited by cultural context as good and evil will differ between cultures and even in time change within a particular culture. Consider when tobacco was first used in this country, smoking was thought to be a pleasurable pastime promoting success and sophistication and actively encouraged and endorsed by society. Today society frowns on smoking it is viewed as detrimental to health and something which should be avoided for the greater good.

It is well documented that smoking is a protagonist in some illnesses such as lung, mouth, throat, bladder cancer and respiratory tract infections among others (Pelucchi et al, 2006) and remains one of the major contributors to death and disease today (Dimond, 2003). Surely this means that the greatest good or moral good would be to prohibit people from smoking? The beneficence would be acting in the best interest of people by taking away what we know today is one of the major causes of lung cancer. The problem with this argument is that to achieve the desired result autonomy would be removed and replaced with a paternalistic doctrine. Another view point comes out of utilitarianism which would advocate a ban on smoking as the greater good would be achieved justifying the loss of autonomy for an individual. Utilitarianism places value on action (Mill, 2007). The problem with utilitarianism is in its use. If we view the health of a nation it is clear that a smoking ban would be the greatest good, but if we apply utilitarianism to an individual enforcing a smoking ban this could be detrimental to their health by taking away what may be their only pleasure and lead to low mood, immobility, social dysfunction and reduced/increased appetite all of which could have a negative impact on their health both physically and mentally to a greater degree than the smoking may have. Utilitarianism in my opinion is incapable of being absolute as its basic foundation being happiness cannot be achieved without knowing sadness. Good health cold be said to be the optimal desire, the problem here is that without knowledge or experience of ill health it would be impossible to put a value on good health. For utilitarianism to be just, a positive value would need to be placed on ill health.

The Kantian philosophy of metaphysics born from Emmanuel Kant a German philosopher argued that ethical dilemmas should be based on the principle that to do evil is bad regardless of the good that may be achieved from the bad act. To demonstrate this in a health context consider conjoined twins sharing a heart likely to die prematurely due to the strain being put on the heart. Kantians would believe that to separate the twins to save one would be an act of evil by denying one twin the chance of life. On the other hand Utilitarian's would believe that to separate the twins would be the greater good as one would survive.

The Nursing and Midwifery Council (NMC) states nurses are responsible for both actions and omissions. In the case of George it would be an act of omission if his smoking was ignored on the basis of respecting his autonomy as the nurse would not be acting in a way to protect the patient's health. Likewise the act of insisting George quite smoking would be wrong on the basis of impinging on George's autonomy. The NMC code of conduct states that its members collaborate/work with others in a way to protect and promote the health and wellbeing of those in their care, their families, carers and wider community. Nurses are obliged to become the patients advocate helping those in their care to access relevant health and social care information and support (NMC, 2008). As long as George is made aware of the consequences relating to his smoking in general and its impact on his present condition and is not incapacitated by pain, is alert, orientated with no mental dysfunction he should be allowed to make his own autonomous choice.

Another argument posed by George's smoking is that of the effects it is having on his family. Second hand smoke causes approximately three thousand deaths a year (Malone, 2008). As we have already seen the NMC states that its members have a responsibility to families and the wider community in addition to their patient. Smoking is a source of air pollution (Hodge, 2004) of which we must all breathe and there for goes against the human right to life (European Commission, Human Rights Act 1998). Again we can look at what philosophers say on the matter. "Satus populi suprema lex esto – the safety of the people is the supreme law" according to the Roman philosopher Cicero (Hodge, 2004). Public health is put at risk by second hand smoke (Adler, 2002). The question now raised is should George be permitted to smoke in his home knowing the risks of second hand smoke could put his family's health under increased risk? (Throckmorton, 2006).

While in practice I have nursed patients both smokers and non smokers, until writing this essay I have paid little mind to patient choice and thought that I was doing the right thing allowing the patient to exercise their autonomous decision to smoke even though I am aware of the effects it can have on their health. Having revisited the NMC code of conduct and researching ethic I feel that my actions were well intended but misplaced as I failed to promote health by informing these patients about the effects of smoking, by doing this I would have been respecting their right to autonomy knowing that their decision to smoke was an informed one.

More interestingly while working on a spinal ward I found that contrary to hospital policy patients were allowed to smoke on the hospital premises, admittedly only in designated areas, being a smoker's shelter and outside the spinal unit. Smoking here was accepted by staff; my opinion on this was that it was out of sympathy as I was told it is allowed as these patients are often in hospital for a long time, sometimes years whereby the hospital becomes their home. I believe the ethics of this choice is based on the life changing disability the patient has had to deal with, whereby the psychological impact of the disability can be more debilitating and traumatic than the disability itself. In this case allowing smoking unchallenged is probably in the patient's best interest as introducing more dilemmas to the patient during this acute stage of their disability could be detrimental to their psychological health and impact on their recovery and relative good health.

In this essay I have identified some ethical dilemmas experienced by healthcare professionals. By looking into what the morals are behind the ethics I have been able to analysis and challenge my own beliefs and put them in context with the NMC guidelines. In relation to the EBL scenario it is clear that an ethical dilemma existed as protecting health and patient autonomy are both pre requisites for the registered nurse. In George's case I have demonstrated how his autonomy can be preserved by making sure he is aware of the facts around his habit and its possible impact on his current health, by doing this the nurse has also fulfilled the NMC requirement to promote health. As there is no legislation that prohibits smoking in private places the nurse is unable to protect the health of George's family and carers arising from second hand smoke inhalation, but is able to promote good health behaviours by informing them about the effects of smoking and information on smoking cessation therapies available.

References

Adier, Greeman, Parker, Kuskowski (2002), Self-Determination and Residents Who Smoke; A Dilemma for the Nursing Home Social Worker, Journal of Social Work In Long Term Car Vol 1(14) pp 19-30, EBSCO host research database SocINDEX [Online], Available at: http://0-web.ebscohost.com.brum.beds.ac.uk/ehost/pdf ?vid=3andhid=102andsid=0c12c3da-263d-41c0-9f5e-355837c9189c%40sessionmgr1102, (Accessed: 2nd June 2009)

Bayer, Stuber (2006), Tobacco Control, Stigma and Public Health: Rethinking the Relations, American Journal of Public Health Vol 96(1) pp47-50, EBSCO host research database Cinhal [Online], Available at: http://0-web.ebscohost.com.brum.beds.ac.uk/ehost/pdf ?vid=9%hid=101andsid=a840b18b-92fd-4c73-80c8-eea4f9b1d363%40sessionmgr109, (Accessed:2nd June 2009)

Dictionary.com (no date), Dictionary.co, [Online] Available at: http://dictionary.reference.com/browse/happi ness, (Accessed 24th June 2009)

Dimond (2003), Smoking and the right to expect a smoke-free environment, British Journal of Nursing Vol 12(5) pp 286-289, EBSCO host research database Cinhal [Online], Available at http://0-web.ebscohost.com.brum.beds.ac.uk/ehost/pdf?vid=4andhid=108andsid=2c0d9aa4-5887-42f7-9fbe-d481aa66a90c%40sessionmgr102, (Accessed: 2nd June 2009)

English Dictionary (2002), Pockets English Dictionary, London, Dorling Kindersley

European Commission (1998) Human Rights Act, Schedule 1 The Articles, Part 1 The Convention, Rights and Freedoms, Article 2 Right to Life, Luxembourg, Office for Official publication of the European Communities, Available [Online} at: http://www.opsi.gov.uk/acts/acts1998/ukpga_19980042_en_3, (Accessed 24th June 2009)

Haddad (1996), Acute care decisions: ethics in action...chemotherapy patient...smoking marijuana, RN 00337021, Vol 59(11)

Hodge, Eber (2004), Tobacco Control Legislation: Tools for Public Health Improvement, The Journal of Law, Medicine and Ethics Vol 32(3) pp 516-523

Jarvie, Malone (2008), Children's Second hand Exposure in Private Homes and Cars: An ethical Analysis, American Journal of Public Health Vol 98(12) pp 2140-2145

Kant (2002), Hill T and Zweig (editor) Groundwork for the Metaphysics of Moral, USA, Oxford University Press

Macniven (1993), Creative Morality, Oxon UK, Routledge

Mill (200and) Roger Crisp (editor) Utilitarianism, USA, Oxford University Press

Nursing and Midwifery Council (2008), Professional code of conduct, Available at: http://www.nmc.uk.org/aArticle.aspx?ArticleI D=3056, (Accessed 2nd June 2009)

Pelucchi, Gallus, Garavello, Bosetti, Vecchia (2006), Cancer risk associated with alcohol and tobacco use: Focus on upper aero-digestive tract and liver, Alcohol Research and Health Vol 29(3) pp 193-198

Readers Panel (2007), A question of responsibility, Nursing Standard Vol 21(27) pp 24

Salladay (2002), Craving a smoke and a beer, Nursing Vol 32(10) pp 78

Throckmorton (2006), Second Hand Smoke and Cancer: Current Evidence and Future Directions in Research, Oncology Nursing Forum Vol 33(2) pp 449-450

www.ingramcontent.com/pod-product-compliance
Lightning Source LLC
Chambersburg PA
CBHW051919170526
45168CB00001B/465